Human Performance Modification
Review of Worldwide Research with a View to the Future

Committee on Assessing Foreign Technology Development in
Human Performance Modification

Division on Engineering and Physical Sciences

Board on Behavioral, Cognitive, and Sensory Sciences
Division on Behavioral and Social Sciences and Education

NATIONAL RESEARCH COUNCIL
OF THE NATIONAL ACADEMIES

THE NATIONAL ACADEMIES PRESS
Washington, D.C.
www.nap.edu

THE NATIONAL ACADEMIES PRESS   500 Fifth Street, NW   Washington, DC 20001

NOTICE: The project that is the subject of this report was approved by the Governing Board of the National Research Council, whose members are drawn from the councils of the National Academy of Sciences, the National Academy of Engineering, and the Institute of Medicine. The members of the committee responsible for the report were chosen for their special competences and with regard for appropriate balance.

This is a report of work supported by Contract HHM402-10-D-0036DO #6 between the Defense Intelligence Agency and the National Academy of Sciences. Any opinions, findings, conclusions, or recommendations expressed in this publication are those of the author(s) and do not necessarily reflect the view of the organizations or agencies that provided support for the project.

International Standard Book Number 13: 978-0-309-26269-9
International Standard Book Number 10: 0-309-26269-0

Limited copies are available from

Division on Engineering and Physical Sciences
National Research Council
500 Fifth Street, NW
Washington, DC 20001
(202) 334-3118

Additional copies are available from

The National Academies Press
500 Fifth Street, NW
Keck 360
Washington, DC 20001
(800) 624-6242 or (202) 334-3313
Internet, http://www.nap.edu

Copyright 2012 by the National Academy of Sciences. All rights reserved.

Printed in the United States of America

THE NATIONAL ACADEMIES
Advisers to the Nation on Science, Engineering, and Medicine

The **National Academy of Sciences** is a private, nonprofit, self-perpetuating society of distinguished scholars engaged in scientific and engineering research, dedicated to the furtherance of science and technology and to their use for the general welfare. Upon the authority of the charter granted to it by the Congress in 1863, the Academy has a mandate that requires it to advise the federal government on scientific and technical matters. Dr. Ralph J. Cicerone is president of the National Academy of Sciences.

The **National Academy of Engineering** was established in 1964, under the charter of the National Academy of Sciences, as a parallel organization of outstanding engineers. It is autonomous in its administration and in the selection of its members, sharing with the National Academy of Sciences the responsibility for advising the federal government. The National Academy of Engineering also sponsors engineering programs aimed at meeting national needs, encourages education and research, and recognizes the superior achievements of engineers. Dr. Charles M. Vest is president of the National Academy of Engineering.

The **Institute of Medicine** was established in 1970 by the National Academy of Sciences to secure the services of eminent members of appropriate professions in the examination of policy matters pertaining to the health of the public. The Institute acts under the responsibility given to the National Academy of Sciences by its congressional charter to be an adviser to the federal government and, upon its own initiative, to identify issues of medical care, research, and education. Dr. Harvey V. Fineberg is president of the Institute of Medicine.

The **National Research Council** was organized by the National Academy of Sciences in 1916 to associate the broad community of science and technology with the Academy's purposes of furthering knowledge and advising the federal government. Functioning in accordance with general policies determined by the Academy, the Council has become the principal operating agency of both the National Academy of Sciences and the National Academy of Engineering in providing services to the government, the public, and the scientific and engineering communities. The Council is administered jointly by both Academies and the Institute of Medicine. Dr. Ralph J. Cicerone and Dr. Charles M. Vest are chair and vice chair, respectively, of the National Research Council.

www.national-academies.org

COMMITTEE ON ASSESSING FOREIGN TECHNOLOGY DEVELOPMENT IN HUMAN PERFORMANCE MODIFICATION

HENDRICK W. RUCK, *Chair,* Human Performance Consulting Group, LLC
JULIE J.C.H. RYAN, *Vice Chair,* George Washington University
ALICE M. AGOGINO (NAE), University of California, Berkeley
DEBRA AUGUSTE, Harvard University
STEVEN G. BOXER (NAS), Stanford University
CHRISTOPER C. GREEN, Wayne State University
HENDRIK F. HAMANN, IBM Research
JAMES C. MILLER, Miller Ergonomics
JOANNA MIRECKI MILLUNCHICK, University of Michigan
DONALD NORMAN (NAE), Nielsen Norman Group
LAURIE ZOLOTH, Northwestern University

Staff

DANIEL E.J. TALMAGE, JR., Study Director
CHERIE CHAUVIN, Senior Program Officer
GREGORY EYRING, Senior Program Officer
SARAH CAPOTE, Research Associate
ZEIDA PATMON, Program Associate

Preface

In fall 2011, the U.S. Army asked the National Research Council to convene a committee to explore the development of capabilities in human performance modification, to review the state of research and identify key players in promising areas of research, and to focus on potential developments that are likely in the next 15 to 25 years.

The Committee on Assessing Foreign Technology Development in Human Performance Modification (see Appendix A) performed a detailed review of available reference material and received briefings from experts in the field, including international researchers (see Appendix B). Preliminary research was conducted by staff from September 2011 to January 2012. The first committee meeting was held on January 19-20, 2012, and the last of three meetings was on March 29-30, 2012 (see Appendix B). The committee compiled draft reports between the last meeting and April 2012, and the report was completed during fall 2012. This report describes fields of current research that the committee found to be most active.

We express our appreciation to the members of the committee for their diligence and dedication in contributing to the study and to the preparation of this report, to the U.S. Army for its sponsorship of the study, and to National Research Council staff members Terry Jaggers, Daniel Talmage, Cherie Chauvin, Sarah Capote, Greg Eyring, and Zeida Patmon for their efforts on behalf of the study.

Hendrick W. Ruck, *Chair*
Julie J.C.H. Ryan, *Vice Chair*
Committee on Assessing Foreign Technology Development in Human Performance Modification

Acknowledgment of Reviewers

This report has been reviewed in draft form by individuals chosen for their diverse perspectives and technical expertise, in accordance with procedures approved by the National Research Council's (NRC's) Report Review Committee. The purpose of this independent review is to provide candid and critical comments that will assist the institution in making its published report as sound as possible and to ensure that the report meets institutional standards for objectivity, evidence, and responsiveness to the study charge. The review comments and draft manuscript remain confidential to protect the integrity of the deliberative process. We wish to thank the following individuals for their review of this report:

Andrew Brown, NAE, Delphi Corporation,
Don Chaffin, NAE, University of Michigan,
Stephen W. Drew, NAE, Drew Solutions,
Mica Endsley, SA Technologies,
Gary Grest, NAE, Sandia National Laboratories,
Douglas Harris, Anacapa Sciences,
Ian McCulloh, U.S. Army,
Martin Moore-Ede, Circadian,
Jonathan Moreno, IOM, University of Pennsylvania Health System, and
Michael Posner, NAS/IOM, University of Oregon.

Although the reviewers listed above have provided many constructive comments and suggestions, they were not asked to endorse the conclusions or recommendations nor did they see the final draft of the report before its release. The review of this report was overseen by Judith L. Swain (IOM), National University of Singapore, who was appointed by the NRC to make certain that an independent review of this report was carried out in accordance with institutional procedures and that all review comments were carefully considered. Responsibility for the final content of this report rests entirely with the authoring committee and the institution.

Contents

SUMMARY   1

1   INTRODUCTION   7
      Background and Rationale for This Study, 7
      Statement of Task and Scope, 7
      Committee Approach, 8
      Report Organization, 9

2   HUMAN COGNITIVE MODIFICATION AS A COMPUTATIONAL PROBLEM   10
      Computation for Human Performance Modification, 10
         Big Data, 10
         Conventional Computers and Current Trends, 12
         Innovations in Computers for Cognitive Information Processing, 14
         Worldwide Research in Cognitive Computing, 16
         Summary Comments, 17
      Computation for Cognitive Enhancement, 17
         Cognitive Artifacts, 17
         Augmented Reality, 18
         Socially Distributed Augmented Reality, 19
         Enhanced Cognitive Performance Through Better Human-Centered Design, 20
         Thoughts on the Concept of Radical Innovation in Cognitive Enhancement, 21
         Cognitive Degradation, 21
         Foreign Research in Cognitive Modification, 22

3   HUMAN PERFORMANCE MODIFICATION AS A BIOLOGICAL PROBLEM   23
      Tissue Engineering, 23
         Worldwide Research, 24
      Fatigue: Judgment and Decision Making, 24
         Worldwide Research, 27

4   HUMAN PERFORMANCE MODIFICATION AS A FUNCTION OF BRAIN-COMPUTER INTERFACES   28
      Brain-Computer Interfaces, 28
         Detection of Electric Signals, 28
         Functional Detection, 29
         Worldwide Research, 30

      Other Kinds of Interfaces, 30
  Nanotechnology for Human Performance Modification, 30
      Worldwide Research, 31

BIBLIOGRAPHY   32

APPENDIXES

A	Biographical Sketches of Committee Members	45
B	Meetings and Speakers	49
C	Acronyms and Abbreviations	52
D	Contextual Issues	53

Summary

The development of technologies to modify natural human physical and cognitive performance is one of increasing interest and concern, especially among military services that may be called on to defeat foreign powers with enhanced warfighter capabilities. *Human performance modification* (HPM) is a general term that can encompass actions ranging from the use of "natural" materials, such as caffeine or khat as a stimulant, to the application of nanotechnology as a drug delivery mechanism or in an invasive brain implant. Although the literature on HPM typically addresses methods that enhance performance, another possible focus is methods that degrade performance or negatively affect a military force's ability to fight.

Advances in medicine, biology, electronics, and computation have enabled an increasingly sophisticated ability to modify the human body, and such innovations will undoubtedly be adopted by military forces, with potential consequences for both sides of the battle lines. Although some innovations may be developed for purely military applications, they are increasingly unlikely to remain exclusively in that sphere because of the globalization and internationalization of the commercial research base.[1]

Based on its review of the literature, the presentations it received, and on its own expertise, the Committee on Assessing Foreign Technology Development in Human Performance Modification chose to focus on three general areas of HPM:

- Human cognitive modification as a computational problem (Chapter 2),
- Human performance modification as a biological problem (Chapter 3), and
- Human performance modification as a function of the brain-computer interface (Chapter 4).

HUMAN COGNITIVE MODIFICATION AS A COMPUTATIONAL PROBLEM

Human perception and performance can be augmented by the use of technological systems that complement and enhance human cognitive abilities: the combined system of the human(s) and the computational tool(s) becomes smarter or more capable than the human alone (Norman, 1993). All functional cognitive systems must have technologies to sense and measure, to process and analyze, and to control or achieve a desired outcome (Norman, 1980). As an example, a system that assists a battle-vehicle operator in maneuvering through rough terrain might record

---

[1] Academic papers reviewed by the committee frequently reflected cooperation between researchers from multiple countries and movement of ideas between university laboratories. Large companies increasingly sponsor global research and development, with laboratories, ideas, and development unrestricted by national borders. Technological development is sped by the global information infrastructure, most notably the Internet, and the rapid worldwide spread of knowledge is normal to the point of being unremarkable.

images with a camera, process the information (for example, categorizing and locating objects in scenes), and alert the operator.

Computation and Human Cognition

The reality of human perception can be modified (augmented) through the use of cognitive artifacts of varied sophistication. Cognitive artifacts are technological systems that complement and enhance human cognitive abilities. A cognitive artifact does not make a person smarter; instead, it is the combined system of the human and the artifact that is smarter or more capable (Norman, 1993). For example, advanced cognitive artifacts can be worn on the body or implanted in various parts of the body and potentially offer enhancement of biological system performance, memory, sensory abilities, and communication.

Augmented reality (AR) has great potential to improve command choices and decisionmaking, with external experts providing relevant information and interpretation from remote and geographically dispersed locations. Another application is enhanced training; through enhanced communication and visualization methods, it is possible to enhance the performance of distributed work teams dramatically. By extension, the integration of nonhuman autonomous components with humans in team-like arrangements could enhance the cognitive performance of groups of humans.

Computational Limitations

The enhancement of cognition by computational means is limited by power demands and architecture design that do not currently support complex cognitive processing. Although information technology (IT) has continued to provide better performance with decreasing power consumption every year, current capabilities are being outpaced by spiraling data and information-processing demands (Izydorczyk, 2010). For example, the IBM Watson is an advanced computing system that "understands" questions in natural language, finds information in relevant sources, determines the confidence level of different options, and responds with factual answers (Ferrucci, 2012). However, Watson's impressive capability for artificial intelligence and cognitive information processing is still far less than the capability of the human brain, which is by comparison orders of magnitude smaller and more efficient. Although advances in data storage and hardware design will improve this situation, computers may need to become more brain-like to meet the requirements of augmented reality.

Reconfigurable computing[2] offers one approach to much more energy efficient, brain-like computers capable of self-learning and adjusting to tasks and requirements without having to be programmed. Such tools for enhancing cognition will require research and development on neuromorphic devices and circuits in which computing elements and memory are "fused" together or finely interleaved (Indiveri et al., 2011). To become brain-like, computers will require dense interconnections between neuron-like computing units. In addition, challenges posed by space constraints for the logical units and by mapping of the neurosynaptic functions of the brain to configuration requirements will have to be overcome. Such developments could fundamentally change the nature of computing, although it might be 15 years or more before real-world applications could be ready.

---

[2]Reconfigurable computing allows the building of intelligent circuits that can be adjusted on the basis of experience and learning.

Worldwide Research

According to the committee's research, the United States currently has a competitive advantage in augmented cognition technology because it leads in the development of human-centered software, although strong research in cognitive computing is performed worldwide. Strong research efforts using reconfigurable computing for neural networks exist in Australia, Ireland, Turkey, and Switzerland. In addition, large international programs, such as the European FACETS (Fast Analog Computing with Emergent Transient States) consortium with participants from seven countries (Austria, France, Germany, Hungary, Sweden, Switzerland, and the United Kingdom), drive research and development for novel neuromorphic computing architectures.

The Importance of Good Design

Machines excel at precise, repetitive operations—tasks for which humans are poorly designed. In contrast, humans excel at tasks requiring flexibility and creativity, and at responding to novel, unexpected situations—tasks in which machines perform poorly. Unfortunately, many computational designs currently do not take advantage of human capabilities and instead force humans to operate by machine rules and logic. With better attention to the well-established principles of human-centered design and human-systems integration, including modeling and simulation of human cognitive performance, there could be a significant enhancement in human cognitive capability with no need for new research or new applications.

Technologies for Degrading Human Cognitive Performance

Although most HPM computational advances are intended to enhance performance, the committee's research identified a class of technology designed to degrade performance. An example has been described by Japanese researchers who have developed a device, using commercial off-the-shelf components, to interfere with and prevent speech production (Kurihara and Tsukada, 2012). In combat or peacekeeping environments, use of such a device could lead to serious consequences by preventing spoken commands, instructions, or assurances intended for friendly or enemy troops, or civilians.[3] Although no additional examples of purposeful degradation of human cognitive capability were uncovered, the potential for such technologies should not be dismissed.

HUMAN PERFORMANCE MODIFICATION AS A BIOLOGICAL PROBLEM

Two primary areas of research and development in HPM as a biological problem were assessed by the committee as having the most likely impact in the next 10-15 years: tissue engineering and mechanisms for addressing fatigue (including sleep patterns).

Tissue Engineering

Tissue engineering can be defined as the use of cells, engineered materials, and suitable biochemical and physiochemical factors to improve or replace biological functions. Success has been achieved in tissues that are thin membranes, that are avascular, or that have high regeneration potential. For example, tissue-engineered skin, cartilage, bone, and corneas have been used clinically (Khademhosseini et al., 2009).

Three approaches to tissue engineering include the conductive approach, which uses a material to provide the structural framework for cell infiltration; the inductive approach, which

---

[3] By contrast, accidental or unintended degradation of human performance can occur with the inappropriate use of devices meant to enhance performance, such as, for example, the use of a cell phone while driving.

uses soluble materials to promote cell infiltration; and the cell-replacement approach, which provides either an allograft (from a donor) or an autologous graft (from the patient) to repair a tissue. Tissue engineering can be used to speed recovery and to improve the quality of the generated tissue. The primary potential application for military purposes is to increase and improve healing processes, thereby returning soldiers to their job duties more quickly. Currently, tissue engineering methods are unable to enhance the normal functioning of healthy tissue. This situation is unlikely to change in the near future because of the substantial challenges involved in organizing large numbers of viable cells.

Worldwide Research

Tissue engineering is a subject of active inquiry throughout the world. The research is being conducted in sports-medicine laboratories, genetic-engineering laboratories, and rehabilitative-surgery centers. The committee found it to be one of the most difficult topics to investigate because it is so vast, varied, and complex. In addition, because the topic involves direct interference in the human body, there are widely differing views worldwide as to what kinds of research are morally acceptable.

Combating the Effects of Fatigue

The negative effects of work-related fatigue on basic psychomotor and cognitive performance are well understood. Physical fatigue manifests itself in deteriorated dexterity, reduced eye-hand coordination, tremors, discomfort, and loss of strength and endurance. The primary contributors to work-related fatigue are long duty hours, inadequate sleep, and disruptions to daily (circadian) rhythms that affect alertness and cognitive performance.

Physical and mental workload are also important determinants of reduced performance due to fatigue (Chaffin et al., 2006). Shift work is especially detrimental, because humans are not wired biologically to work at night. In the pre-dawn hours, the metabolic rate begins to drop toward its circadian low point, and complex biological mechanisms in the brain that generate sleep are at their most powerful.

Fatigue has been studied extensively, and models have been incorporated into formalized fatigue risk-management plans. The accrued knowledge has been used to optimize operational plans and to inform the choice of shift and movement scheduling. New technologies that have been developed to detect and manage fatigue range from timed use of pharmacologic agents, such as modafinil, to highly precise light treatment devices. The integration of the technologies into management of human resources may affect the functional effectiveness of units that operate in extreme situations, such as long shifts, rotating shifts, and quick deployments across many time zones.

There is research funding for some knowledge gaps, including those related to the effects of fatigue on team cognitive performance and the elucidation of phenotype and genotype for sleep and fatigue traits. Some knowledge gaps without research funding are related to nontherapeutic effects of transcranial stimulation on sleep and psychomotor performance, interactive effects of automation and fatigue on human operators' cognitive skills, and the effects of fatigue on higher-level cognitive constructs, such as naturalistic decision making, risk taking, and situation awareness.

In the next 5 to 10 years, top-down fatigue-risk management systems will become commonplace in 24/7 operations, as will the practice of removing sleep debt before critical operations. In the next 10 to 15 years, pre-travel adjustment of the circadian rhythm will be routine, and on-duty napping during 24/7 and nighttime operations will become an accepted practice.

The committee also found that genetic analysis of individuals with unique sleep patterns has important potential for military operations. This category includes short sleepers, those susceptible to sleep deprivation or restriction, and people who experience unique circadian rhythm effects. Large-scale screenings are underway to identify genes that regulate sleep, and sleep circuitries and functions are being investigated at a molecular level. If a military force could remain fully functional with less sleep than its enemy, the implications for military effectiveness could be significant.

Worldwide Research

The results obtained by the committee indicate that the European Union is the leader in the field of fatigue research, with the United States, Australia, and Japan providing extensive contributions as well. Shift work in railroad operations, similar to military operations whose 24-hour demands encourage irregular schedules based on the clock, has been studied extensively in Europe and Japan. Only recently has the United States begun to fund similar research to better understand the physical, cognitive, and other effects of irregularly scheduled work. Additional countries conducting notable research include Brazil, Canada, Iceland, New Zealand, Norway, Singapore, and South Korea.

HUMAN PERFORMANCE MODIFICATION AS A FUNCTION OF THE BRAIN-COMPUTER INTERFACE

Brain-Computer Interfaces

Brain-computer interfaces (BCIs) involve direct communication of neural signals with an external device. A large body of research is concerned with the ability to detect and translate neural activity and to direct it to control a machine and thereby enhance human performance (Brunner et al., 2011). The most common application is in the realm of rehabilitative medicine. For example, neural implants that enable a disabled person to control a wheelchair, prosthesis, or voice simulator have been developed (Rebsamen et al., 2010; Bell et al., 2008; Brumberg and Guenther, 2010). Conversely, electronic signals may be used to stimulate portions of the brain to induce a particular motor response, although this effect has been demonstrated only in animals (Arfin et al., 2009; Nuyujukian et al., 2011). Although potential applications for performance enhancement may develop in the future, current BCIs are slower and less accurate than the normal human function they are meant to replace.

Critical to the successful use/operation of brain-computer interfaces is the identification of brain regions activated during particular processes. Recently, electroencephalogram (EEG) spectra obtained using neural probes implanted into a subject's brain have been successfully reconstructed as sounds heard by the subject. Future research will seek to extend this capability to analyze EEG spectra of thoughts and convert them to speech. This is an exciting advance that could lead to individuals regaining their lost ability to speak.

Role of Nanotechnology

The implementation of BCIs and many other HPM technologies is enabled by nanotechnology, which can be instantiated in a wide variety of technologies and fields relevant to HPM, including electronics, microelectromechanical systems, energy harvesting and storage devices/systems, and biomedicine. Especially intriguing for HPM is the use of nanotechnology for biointerfaces—materials, smaller than cells, that could possibly interact directly with the body on a biological level. For example, subdermal nanoparticles inserted into the body could enhance sensory perception (Cash and Clark, 2010).

A more invasive use of nanotechnology for HPM is in the development of neural implants. These devices are placed directly into the brain to detect electric signaling (Navarro et al., 2005). To increase the signal-to-noise ratio and the resolution, the probes have to be on the same scale as the neurons that they monitor, that is, with a size of a few micrometers. Furthermore, they must be made of materials that are biocompatible and that produce as little damage and scarring in the surrounding tissue as possible. Sophisticated nanomaterials are being developed to achieve these characteristics (Zhang and Webster, 2009).

Worldwide Research

The committee's literature search suggested that non-U.S. entities are more active in such research on cognitive function, with international players including Israel, Germany, Japan, and the Netherlands. Taiwan and South Korea have research infrastructure and expertise in this area as well, and China has also shown interest. Despite a great deal of progress, however, how the human brain functions is still largely unknown, and it seems unlikely that human performance can be significantly enhanced via BCIs in the near term.

CONCLUDING THOUGHTS

It is clear that human performance modification—both for enhancement and degradation of capabilities—is a subject of active research in all the technologically developed countries and regions of the world. The span of research is enormous, ranging from sports-related research to worker-enhancement research, to military applications. And the potential for crossover applications in each category is high. For example, research in injury recovery and physical performance enhancement, now mostly in the sports-research sector, clearly has applicability to military force development and maintenance.

The committee noted that the sheer breadth of the scope of inquiry is staggering, from nanotechnology to genetic engineering to manipulating normal human processes (such as healing or fatigue). Predicting where each will go is difficult; predicting or even imagining the interactions, cross-applications, and unintended consequences borders on the impossible. One need only look at today's human performance modifications that were not even dreamed about 20 years ago: wireless pacemakers that are monitored over the Internet, massively multiplayer on-line games that are used for tactics and training, and global groupware that enables geographically distributed teamwork. These examples show how one development—the commodification of the Internet backbone—enabled huge changes.

Although some technologies are exotic and require specialized infrastructure and knowledge, such as nanotechnology and genetic engineering, others (perhaps most) do not require such infrastructure and can be pursued with fairly minimal investments. This situation makes it problematic to monitor the state of HPM technology development. The complexity of the field requires monitoring of the entire technology ecosystem (see Appendix D) associated with any element of an application.

Finally, because of its very nature, HPM technology development will be influenced by differing legal norms, cultural values, and social mores in different parts of the world. It is a form of bias to assume that the methods and approaches used in one's own geographic area are the same as those used in other areas. And even within a given country, there may be differences with regard to social mores, philosophies, and legal constraints. Two examples that illustrate the point are agriculture research involving genetically modified organisms and stem-cell research. In some parts of the world the former is fully acceptable and the latter less so, and vice versa in other parts. Any analysis of potential developments in HPM must be attuned to these cultural influences.

1
Introduction

BACKGROUND AND RATIONALE FOR THIS STUDY

The development of technologies that expand and change natural human physical and cognitive performance is of increasing interest and concern. There is a long history of humans modifying both body and mind in order to modify performance; examples range from the ingestion of materials derived from nature such as caffeine or the leaves of the coca plant (from which cocaine is derived) to training regimens, electronic stimulation, and ergonomic system design. Human performance modification (HPM) practices continue today with such products as energy drinks, brain-training video games, and specialized nutritional regimens for athletes, as well as modeling of individual performance for analysis and enhancement.

With the growth of increasingly sophisticated scientific capabilities in medicine, biology, electronics, and computation, the ability to modify human performance has expanded and changed. Current avenues of research span a wide array of sciences and technologies, including brain physiology and function, genetic modification, and nanotechnology. The resulting innovations will undoubtedly find their way into military forces, for good or for ill. Some innovations may even be developed for purely military use, although they are increasingly unlikely to remain exclusively in that sphere because of the globalization of the commercial research base (NRC, 2005; NAS-NAE-IOM, 2007, 2010). The committee explored how these technologies are developing, both from the standpoint of understanding what other entities may be doing, and for applications relevant to the U.S. armed forces.

STATEMENT OF TASK AND SCOPE

The statement of ask for this study is shown in Box 1-1. Given the broad scope of the HPM field, the committee had to be selective in terms of the topics it investigated in depth. The sponsor also provided some guidance by expressing interest not only in technologies for enhancing the performance of both individual humans and teams, but also in technologies aimed at degrading their performance. Based on this guidance, its review of the literature, the presentations it received, and on its own expertise, the committee chose three general areas of focus:

- Human cognitive modification as a computational problem,
- Human performance modification as a biological problem, and
- Human performance modification as a function of the brain-computer interface.

> **Box 1-1**
> **Statement of Task**
>
> The National Research Council will form an ad hoc committee to focus on developmental capabilities in the general area of human performance modification. The committee will perform an initial review of the literature, select the most promising areas, and identify the lead players (state or non-state) in those areas. Areas of investigation include biotechnology, brain-computer interfaces, cognitive enhancement, electronics, nanotechnology, and neural implants. This does not preclude additional areas uncovered during the course of the study. The committee will exclude conventional pharmaceuticals and exoskeletons per the sponsor's direction.
> The committee will then:
>
> 1) Identify and describe the technical maturity of research efforts emphasizing the top non-U.S. players;
> 2) Describe the research and development environment with a particular focus on governmental policy;
> 3) Characterize the developmental timeline for each of the technologies;
> 4) Assess the implications of the technology development in the 15-25 year timeframe;
> 5) Offer findings or conclusions on issues such as possible scientific-technology "mismatches," research or technology "breakthroughs," or identify "gaps" in scientific findings or technology.

Reviewers of this report pointed out a number of worthy topics that were not considered here, either because they do not have a strong technology component or because of the committee's limited time and resources:

- Virtual reality (though augmented reality is discussed),
- Ergonomics,
- Human simulation models, including cognitive models,
- Social modification of human performance, including better leadership and management,
- Enhancements in group cognition, and
- Implanted devices.

COMMITTEE APPROACH

For each of the HPM technologies selected above, the committee discusses the technological maturity (Task 1), implications (Task 4), and research needs (Task 5). To the extent it could, the committee comments on the expected development timelines for the technologies (Task 3), although forecasting technology development is notoriously difficult (see Appendix D).

There were a number of challenges encountered in addressing the activities of non-U.S. players (Task 1) and government policy (Task 2). It quickly became apparent that the globalization of research, both in academe and in industry, precluded a nation-by-nation approach. Academic papers of interest commonly featured cooperation between researchers in multiple countries and movement of ideas among university laboratories. Companies large enough to sponsor research and development are increasingly global and have laboratories in many countries. The flow of intellectual activities is sped by the global information infrastructure, most notably the Internet.

The committee's literature search relied on published, unclassified work, available in the English language. However, it is likely that much research in this field is not being published or is not available in English, and may be classified. The committee did receive briefings from multiple foreign researchers and did discuss foreign priorities, but this partial information did not provide a definitive picture of either U.S. or foreign government priority setting and policy in research on human performance modification (Task 2).

As an interesting aside, the committee noted that in keeping with previous trends associated with science fiction serving as an inspiration for research and development efforts, today's research appears to be strongly influenced by contemporary entertainment products, including movies, books, games, and anime. In particular, the committee noted that such concepts as the Borg from the *Star Trek*[1] series were invoked as referents during several of the data-collection efforts, as were the X-Men[2] and the Terminator[3] from the movies of the same name. However, the committee also noted that such science fiction creates many false impressions of what science might be capable of allowing humans to perform. In addition to reviewing academic peer-reviewed literature, the committee and staff also put significant effort into researching popular science and considering the efficacy of the reported results against basic scientific limitations. This research and the committee's observations are presented in Appendix D.

REPORT ORGANIZATION

Chapter 2 discusses several topics under the general heading of human cognitive modification as a computational problem, including applications of augmented reality. Chapter 3 explores two aspects of HPM viewed as a biological problem: human tissue engineering and fatigue research. Several topics under the general heading of HPM as a function of the brain-computer interface, including applications of nanotechnology, are discussed in Chapter 4.

Appendixes A-C provide committee biographies, a list of meetings and presenters, and a list of acronyms, respectively. Important contextual issues affecting technology development are discussed in Appendix D, including relevant differences in cultures and value systems among technology developers, technology ecosystem requirements, and the identification of required scientific or technological breakthroughs.

---

[1] Paramount Pictures, Star Trek: First Contact, 1996.
[2] Marvel Comics; see http://marvel.com/universe/X-Men.
[3] Helmsdale Pictures, Terminator, 1984, distributed by Orion Pictures; see http://www.imdb.com/title/tt0088247/.

2
Human Cognitive Modification as a Computational Problem

COMPUTATION FOR HUMAN PERFORMANCE MODIFICATION

Human performance modification (HPM) can be considered as an application of cognitive technologies in which different components have to work as an integrated system. The components and the system architecture and design are determined by the specifics of the HPM application. At a high level, all functional cognitive systems must have technologies to sense and measure, to process and analyze, and to control or achieve a desired outcome (Norman, 1980). For example, a system that assists a battle-vehicle operator in maneuvering through rough terrain might record images with a camera, process the information (for example, categorizing and locating objects in scenes), and alert the operator.

Many of today's simpler information-processing requirements for HPM are met by conventional computing technologies, which are not discussed here. In discussing more advanced computing concepts, the committee does not distinguish between different forms of computing implementation (such as wearable computing versus stationary systems) but rather focuses on important trends in information technology (IT) development and research for both military and commercial computing applications. The trends include the challenge of managing what is referred to as big data, the need for alternative computational architectures, and an increasingly close coupling of humans and machines (as in augmented reality).

Big Data

One of the greatest challenges for realizing more complex and advanced HPM applications in the cognitive realm is posed by the need for processing large amounts of often unstructured data, such as speech or video. In recent years, the notion of big data has emerged to describe this trend. More and more datasets are collected, and their size and complexity are not only well beyond human cognitive capabilities, but also often beyond today's computer information-processing capabilities. The current projection of data growth is 40 percent per year, meaning that data volume would double every 2 years (Manyika et al., 2011; Miller, 1956; Bohn and Short, 2010; Simon, 1971; Maguire et al., 2007).

The projection on data growth is informed by the trend toward collecting data on everything, with numerous commercial ventures attempting to contain all the data in the world,[1] along with intelligence agencies and other government agencies. Data mining, or machine learning, is now a big business. Data fusion, which originally meant the combining of data gathered with different kinds of sensors, now means the combining of data of various sorts from different databases and repositories. The data are often in incompatible formats with different categorization rules and standards and different semantics, but these limitations are being overcome. The current approach

---

[1] See, for example, http://www.factual.com.

of using structured databases to provide reasonable answers to queries is being supplanted by emerging technologies that are able to interpret, address, and integrate unstructured, natural data by using unstructured, natural-language queries that more closely reflect human language processing and analytic approaches.

Big data as a concept has implications for the demands placed on humans to understand rapidly growing bodies of information and for the possibility of augmenting human cognition through breakthroughs in computer-based processing. Sensor suites used in science, military applications, and complex system operations can flood a human operator with data and result in a decrease in system performance due to cognitive overload. Computational systems to augment human cognition are being developed to address this problem. Research is addressing the best ways for people to interact with and control systems that are increasingly complex, but the research seems to be limited in its generalizability. An example is the "optimal" cockpit in military aviation. Despite nearly 100 years of experience, the optimal design of cockpit displays, controls, and automation tradeoffs is still controversial. The question of how much a human should be involved in the operation of a system will be critical as HPM technologies associated with big data continue to evolve.

Big data has been made possible by a series of IT advancements, including the reduction in the cost of data storage and computing, the emergence of the Internet, widespread deployment of video and other sensor technologies, advanced computer networks, cloud-computing technologies, social networks, and smart phones. Although the notion of big data is discussed primarily in the context of commercial and business applications, where it promises great advances in productivity, it is clear that big data technologies will be critical for—and beneficial to—military-oriented HPM applications.

Managing big data poses substantial challenges, and the following discussion assumes that organizations, countries, or other entities that make the most progress toward solving the fundamental scalability challenges associated with big data and cognitive information processing will have the best basis for developing game-changing HPM applications.

Scientists and engineers working in the IT sector are making—and will continue to make—substantial improvements in many areas, including leveraging high-speed networking, parallel and cluster computer programming, cloud computing, machine learning, advanced data-storage technologies, continued scaling of Moore's law (which states that the number of transistors on an integrated circuit board will double about every 2 years), and security technologies. However, as discussed in more detail below, the current trajectory does not support future computing requirements, especially as it applies to big data and cognitive information processing. Even today, serious challenges are evident in relation to scalability and sustainability of the current trends. Three examples illustrate the problems: unsustainable energy needs, the explosion of data produced, and the current inefficiency of computing solutions that mimic human intelligence.

Energy needs are a recognized challenge. Although IT technology continues to provide better performance with less power consumption every year, it is now well established that past advances have not been able to keep pace with information-processing demands (Izydorczyk, 2010). Specifically, a study estimated total U.S. data-center energy consumption in 2005 to be about 1.2 percent of total U.S. consumption, which is an increase of 15 percent from 2000 (Koomey, 2007). Total power consumption for IT is still low compared with other sectors, but the growth rate of 15 percent (that is, doubling every 5 years) is alarming and suggests that the continued expansion of IT is not sustainable. Clearly, improved IT energy efficiency will be critical to addressing the sustainability of growth. Major innovations will be required to scale big data technologies to levels where they will provide the anticipated benefits (U.S. Code, 2008).

The explosion of data is also a recognized challenge. The problem is illustrated by the new radio telescope developed by the Square Kilometer Array (SKA) Consortium (Crosby, 2012). The telescope will produce 1 exabyte (1 billion gigabytes) of data every day. To put that into context, the whole Internet today handles about 0.5 exabyte per day. It would be naïve to assume that a viable exabyte computer can be built without major technology innovations. The innovations will need to include new architectures, new approaches to software, and new hardware technologies, including advanced accelerators, 3-D stacked chips for more energy-efficient computing, novel optical interconnect technologies to optimize data transfer and communication, and new high-performance storage systems based on next-generation tape systems and novel phase-change memory (IBM, 2012).

Finally, mimicking of human intelligence in today's computing environment is recognized as inefficient. The IBM Watson computer is arguably one of the most advanced computing systems that specializes in natural human language and provides specific answers to complex questions at high speeds (Ferrucci, 2012). Specifically, the system "understands" questions in natural language, finds information in relevant sources, and determines the confidence of different options and responses with factual answers. Watson applies technologies from different fields, such as machine learning, natural-language processing, information retrieval, knowledge presentation, and hypothesis generation. In February 2011, the Watson computer won the game of Jeopardy against two all-time champions. But the cost of such achievement is high: the system consists of 90 Linux servers, 2,880 Power7 processor cores (3.55 GHz), and almost 16 terabytes (16,000 gigabytes) of random-access memory. The computer comes in four racks and weighs more than 10,000 pounds, needs 25 tons of cooling equipment, and consumes around 100 kW of electricity (the consumption of 40–50 households).

Although the Watson computer is one of the most impressive instances of artificial intelligence and cognitive information processing, it is far from the capabilities of the human brain, which by comparison uses only a few watts of electricity, weighs around 3 pounds, and fits into the palms of two hands. Specifically, given today's technology trajectory, which improves power performance of computing systems by 25-30 percent per year, the Watson computer would still consume about 1,000 W in 15 years—still far from the power consumption of a human brain (apart from the fact that the human brain can do much more than the Watson computer).

It is clear from the three challenges discussed above that innovations in computing infrastructure are required if important advances are to be made. To provide context, the committee describes the current computational structure briefly below and then discusses needed changes.

Conventional Computers and Current Trends

The fundamental reason that the human brain is far superior to any of today's computers is that the brain operates in a completely different manner from a conventional computer. Conventional computers are commonly referred to as von Neumann machines; they were developed over 40 years ago for the applications and programming problems that were relevant then. A distinct feature of von Neumann machines is that they share a bus between a central processing unit (CPU) and memory. Information cannot be exchanged back and forth between the CPU and the memory at the same time, and this makes the bus a bottleneck—commonly referred as the von Neumann bottleneck (Backus, 1978). Before an instruction or word can be sent through the bus, the CPU must know the address, which had to be sent before. The von Neumann architecture results in an instruction-at-a-time processing approach, substantially unlike that of the human brain, which uses a massively parallel system of slower processing units (neurons) that are connected by weights.[2] The weights are called synapses; each neuron has about 103 synapses. The strengths of the synapses are constantly modified by the learning experience and memory. A

---

[2] It should be noted that the comparison between the human brain and the von Neumann architecture is recognized as limited in applicability; other characteristics of the human brain slow responses in some circumstances, as in socially constrained environments.

human brain has about 10^{10} neurons (processing units) working in the kilohertz regime, whereas a CPU might have only four cores working in the gigahertz regime.

Although deficiencies of the von Neumann architecture have been known for a long time, the limitations have become evident only recently because the continued increase in clock frequency of microprocessors effectively hid the impact of the von Neumann bottleneck. In the past, faster transistor performance, achieved by shrinking the transistor device, offset the effects of the von Neumann bottleneck. With transistor sizes in the 20-nm regime, fundamental limitations have emerged whereby device performance is governed by finite size (or quantum) effects. As a consequence, whereas in the past transistors and microprocessors could be made faster without increasing power consumption (a fundamental feature of Dennard's scaling laws), this is no longer possible (Dennard et al., 1974). The phenomenon is generally referred to as the power wall (Meenderinck and Juurlink, 2009). To continue to provide computational performance improvements at constant power, industry has moved quickly to multicore processors and accelerators (Iancu et al., 2010; Clark et al., 2005). That approach has delayed the impact of the power wall, but the multicore approach is not a "silver bullet."

As a consequence of the trend toward multicore processing, another challenge has emerged: how to support each core with enough memory. Most of today's multicore microprocessor chip space is memory or cache (memory wall) (Zia et al., 2009). In addition, the use of—and reliance on—specific accelerators to provide more performance has made the CPU less general. The variety of circuits and boards is exploding, and with them the size of the teams required for research and development; all this adds cost to the design and building of computing systems.

The current trends in the industry toward multicore processors, cell processors, general-purpose processors (GPUs), accelerators, and so on, can be viewed as "incremental" stages toward a non–von Neumann computing paradigm (Gschwind, 2007; Nickolls and Dally, 2010). These trends are expected to continue over the next 10-15 years. Nevertheless, major technology innovations would be required in the next 10-15 years to produce a Watson-like supercomputer that would be hand-held and have a footprint and power consumption comparable with those of a human brain. Such a device would have a game-changing impact, not only in the commercial arena for big data processing, but also for military and HPM applications.

Thus, the IT industry, driven by big data requirements and power efficiency needs, is at a critical juncture. Three scenarios can be envisioned for the next 15 years: business as usual, computing with low-voltage devices, and neuromorphic computing (see Table 2-1). These scenarios will most likely coexist in parallel, but also compete against one another. Each succeeding scenario is more disruptive to the status quo but promises greater improvements in IT energy efficiency and thus has more potential for cognitive computing applications.

It is expected that the "business as usual" scenario will continue to play an important role using (basically) today's von Neumann architectures in which computations are carried out sequentially under program control by repeatedly fetching an instruction, decoding it, and executing it. Expected improvements include technologies for improving system integration (such as 3-D silicon, silicon photonics, storage-class memory, and so on) and new nanoscale devices (such as nanowires and carbon electronics).

As an alternative to the first scenario, new architectures (von Neumann and non–von Neumann) could emerge that could leverage very low-voltage (but also lower-performing) device technologies. This scenario would allow many more devices on a computer chip than today (hundreds of billions) while improving the energy efficiency of computation. It could include such technologies as spintronics.

The third scenario involves reconfigurable computing to realize non–von Neumann machines. It might lead to much more energy-efficient, brain-like computers without programming. These computers would feature self-learning, and would adjust to tasks and requirements with enhanced cognitive capabilities. As will become clear, this direction will require research and development on new neuromorphic devices and circuits in which computing elements and memory are "fused" together or finely interleaved (Indiveri et al., 2011). Because this scenario would fundamentally change the nature of computing, it might be more than 15 years before such technologies are ready for real-world applications.

TABLE 2-1 Computing Technology Scenarios

Technology Scenario	Key Technologies	Programming	Efficiency Gains and Cognitive capabilities	Architecture
1—Business as Usual	3-D packaging, storage-class memory, silicon photonics, nanowires, carbon electronics	Computing with programming	Moderate	Von Neumann
2—Computing with low-voltage devices	Low-voltage devices, spintronics	Some programming	Medium	Von Neumann and non–von Neumann
3—Neuromorphic computing	New neuromorphic circuits, phase-change memory, memristors	Computing with no programming	High	Non–von Neumann

Innovations in Computers for Cognitive Information Processing

Some types of computer hardware (optical, analog, and quantum computers) are better suited than others to realizing a non–von Neumann computer architecture. Such architectures may use quantum and nonquantum information-processing methods. Research on alternative non–von Neumann computers is active around the world. The challenges facing the development of brain-like computers are enormous: very dense interconnect requirements between the neuron-like computing units, space constraints for the logical units, the analog nature of the neurosynaptic functions of the brain, and complex configuration requirements.

There have been important advances in reconfigurable computing in recent years, particularly in embedded systems (Hartenstein, 1997). Unlike hard-wired technology in the form of application-specific integrated circuits (ASICs) or CPUs, reconfigurable computing uses software-programmed logic. A circuit is flexible and is mapped to the application. Even more important, the circuit can be changed over the life of the system or application. In essence, reconfigurable computing allows the building of intelligent circuits that can be adjusted on the basis of experience and learning. The most common form of reconfigurable computing uses field-programmable gate arrays (FPGAs), which have an array of logic units. The functionality of each of these units can be set by programmable configurations. The connections between the elements or logical units are also programmable, and this makes an FPGA as flexible as software. FPGAs are well suited for artificial neural networks (NNs) or spiking neural networks (SNNs) because of their parallel and distributed network of relatively simple processing units, which can be dynamically adapted as to exploit concurrency and rapidly reconfigured to adapt to weights and topologies of an NN (Ghani et al., 2006; Glackin et al., 2005; Upegui et al., 2005; Pearson et al., 2007; Ros et al., 2006).

Substantial performance improvements in selected cognitive computing tasks have been demonstrated with FPGA technology, although FPGA technology specifications are poor by comparison to ASICs (Hartenstein, 1997). The reason for the good performance with "bad" technology specifications is that effective integration density of FPGAs can be much higher by including a domain-specific mix of hardware and configured logical units within the FPGA fabrics. For example, the dataflow computer (a hardware architecture that uses FPGAs) is designed to utilize convolutional neural networks for general recognition and classification tasks, and can be applied to object recognition, face detection, or robot navigation (Farabet et al., 2009). The researchers demonstrated a system for providing "real-time detection, categorization and localization of objects in complex scenes, while consuming only 10 W," which was "about about ten times less than a laptop computer, and producing speedups of up to 100 times in real-world applications" (Farabet et al., 2011).

Although the dataflow-computer example shows potential for useful HPM applications, real game-changers for scalable NN hardware implementations face fundamental challenges. Much more efficient and smaller implementations of synaptic junctions and neuron interconnects have to be developed. For example, existing FPGA implementation limits the density of synapses as they are mapped onto logic elements of the FPGA. These logic elements are still much too big and too power-hungry to be able to scale the technology (Maguire et al., 2007). Another challenge is presented by the Manhattan-style routing structures, which cannot accommodate the very high levels of neuron interconnectivity as the numbers of neurons grow. To be scalable, the numbers of interconnections and the associated power consumption have to be addressed as more "neurons" are realized on a chip. Similar issues exist in other implementations that use system-on-chip technologies. Alternative approaches using network-on-chip concepts are being researched and promise improvements because the higher levels of connectivity can be provided without incurring a large interconnect-to-device area ratio (Harkin et al., 2009; Maguire et al., 2007).

Other exploratory approaches intended to deal with the current challenges use silicon-based neuromorphic chips (Indiveri et al., 2011). Some implementations exploit the biophysical equivalence between the transport of ions in biological channels and charge transfer in transistor channels. It has been shown that it is possible to build biophysically faithful silicon implementations of different spiking neurons (Morgan et al., 2009; Hynna and Boahen, 2009). However, the circuits are very large and complex even if advanced silicon technology is exploited. More compact circuits have been demonstrated with the goal of connecting large numbers of them on a single chip (Yu and Cauwenberghs, 2010). A common application of the very compact, basic spiking circuits is their use in neuromorphic vision sensors (Schemmel et al., 2008). Research and development aimed at combining analog and digital circuits optimally are going on.

In the most prominent implementation of neuromorphic circuits, the SyNAPSE (System of Neuromorphic Adaptive Plastic Scalable Electronics) project uses digital circuits that exploit the scalability, noise characteristics, and robustness of silicon technology (Olsson and Häfliger, 2008). Digital neuron circuits are supported by transposable static random-access memory arrays that share learning circuits to enable efficient on-chip learning of cognitive tasks. In this architecture, the number of learning circuits grows only with the number of neurons, and this is a clear advantage (Seo et al., 2011). Neurons are connected with a crossbar fanout. An initial configurable chip was demonstrated with 256 neurons and 64 K binary synapses; it was built in 45-nm silicon-on-insulator complementary metal oxide–semiconductor technology. The power efficiency of the chip was optimized by using a near-threshold event-driven operation.

Interesting device options have been proposed to mimic plasticity, which is the neurons' ability, through their synapses, to have memory, learn, adapt, and evolve in response to their environment. For example, phase-change memory materials have been proposed to perform neurosynaptic functions (Modha and Singh, 2010). Phase-change materials are considered to be a memory technology that replaces charge-based storage in the semiconductor industry. In contrast with charge-based storage, they allow nonbinary and nonvolatile information processing. Another approach is based on a memristive device, which was initially proposed in 1976 (Rusu, 2007).

Like a phase-change device, the memristor can remember its stimulation history without power (Chua and Kang, 1976).

Worldwide Research in Cognitive Computing

Research in cognitive computing is a very active and emerging field around the world; many groups and institutions are involved. It can be assumed that most innovations in this field will become pervasive and generally available, especially in light of the commoditization and globalization trends of the IT industry. A number of foreign groups are using FPGAs and reconfigurable computing for neural networks:

- Advanced Computing Research Centre (University of South Australia, Adelaide, Australia),
- Bio-Inspired Electronics and Reconfigurable Computing Research Group (National University of Ireland, Galway, Ireland),
- Department of Computer Engineering (Kocaeli University, Izmit, Turkey),
- Intelligent Systems Research Centre (University of Ulster, Magee Campus, Derry, Northern Ireland),
- Institute of Neuroinformatics (University of Zurich and ETH Zurich, Switzerland), and
- School of Information Technology and Electrical Engineering (University of Queensland, Brisbane, Queensland, Australia).

Other countries also have large programs for the development of new forms of computing. For example, the European FACETS (Fast Analog Computing with Emergent Transient States) consortium was created to drive research and development for novel neuromorphic computing architectures. The consortium includes participants in seven countries (Austria, France, Germany, Hungary, Sweden, Switzerland, and the United Kingdom). Leading research groups in this field around the world include:

- Institute of Neuroinformatics (University of Zurich and ETH Zurich, Switzerland),
- Integrated Systems Group (University of Edinburgh, UK),
- Institute of Microelectronics of Seville (National Microelectronics Center, Seville, Spain),
- Department of Electronic and Computer Engineering (Hong Kong University of Science and Technology, Hong Kong, China),
- School of Electrical Engineering and Telecommunications (University of New South Wales, Sydney, Australia),
- School of Electrical and Electronic Engineering (University of Manchester, Manchester, UK),
- Department of Informatics (University of Oslo, Oslo, Norway),
- Laboratoire de l'Intégration du Matériau au Système (Bordeaux University and IMS-CNRS Laboratory, Bordeaux, France),
- Kirchhoff Institute for Physics (University of Heidelberg, Heidelberg, Germany),
- Department of Computer Science and Engineering (Shanghai Jiao Tong University, Shanghai, China),
- Department of Computer Science and Technology (Tsinghua University, Beijing, China),
- School of Electronics and Information Engineering (Tongji University, Shanghai, China),
- Department of Electrical Engineering and Information Systems (University of Tokyo, Tokyo, Japan), and

- Chinese Academy of Sciences, China.

Summary Comments

Today's computers are limited by "an-instruction-at-a-time" architecture (the von Neumann paradigm) and so are not designed to support complex cognitive processing tasks. The emergence of big data will drive innovation to non–von Neumann computers, which will have enhanced cognitive computing capabilities. The IT industry has taken first steps toward non–von Neumann computers by using GPUs, accelerators, multiprocessors, and so on.

Even today's most powerful computers are many orders of magnitude away from the cognitive processing capabilities of a human brain. Fundamental innovations in hardware, software, and programming languages are required to make more substantial progress toward a computer that has brain-like efficiency and cognitive capabilities.

Reconfigurable computing (realizable with FPGAs) has made progress toward more advanced cognitive processing capabilities and will continue to evolve. However, there are substantial challenges (related to power, size, and interconnectivity) that must be overcome before reconfigurable computing can mimic more advanced SNNs. New forms of neuromorphic chips and devices are being explored to mimic brain circuits. Most near-term HPM applications will leverage off-the-shelf, commodity computers.

COMPUTATION FOR COGNITIVE ENHANCEMENT

It is important to distinguish research from practice. Research takes place in scientific laboratories and, in general, is done by academic, industrial, or government laboratories. Research helps to develop understanding of technologies and procedures, but laboratory research is often ill suited to commercial applications, being too specialized, insufficiently robust, and often prohibitively expensive.

Practical applications are usually developed by technology incubators, startups, or companies, although applications with military implications are often developed by military laboratories. Technology development is often held as a closely guarded secret. In the commercial realm, that is necessary to maintain a competitive advantage. In military domains, it is held as a secret for similar reasons: to maintain an advantage and to keep adversaries from developing powerful new techniques.

There are several potential technologies and methods for cognitive enhancement, including the use of cognitive artifacts and the integration of many technologies to create augmented reality (AR) capabilities.

Cognitive Artifacts

Cognitive artifacts are things or technological systems that complement and enhance human cognitive abilities. Just as a car makes a human faster and a drill or crane enhances a human's physical capabilities, cognitive artifacts enhance human mental processing capabilities. Writing is an example of a cognitive artifact that enhances memory, communication, education, and thinking. More advanced cognitive artifacts, such as smart phones and cochlear implants, are portable. A cognitive artifact does not make a person smarter: it is the combination of the human and the artifact that is smarter or more capable than the human alone (Norman, 1993). The effects of cognitive artifacts can be observed in enhanced methods of training and in enhanced communication and visualization methods, which make it possible to enhance the performance of distributed work teams dramatically. Distributed work teams may include nonhuman components: sensors, teleoperated systems, computational devices, and autonomous robots ("automatons"). The largest benefits of cognitive enhancement will probably emerge in distributed work team concepts.

Cognitive artifacts can take on numerous forms, but it is convenient to categorize them along a mobility continuum from stationary external devices to mobile external devices to devices implanted in the body. It is also useful to understand the degree of virtuality of a device, from complete virtual reality to various degrees of augmented reality (see Figure 2-1).

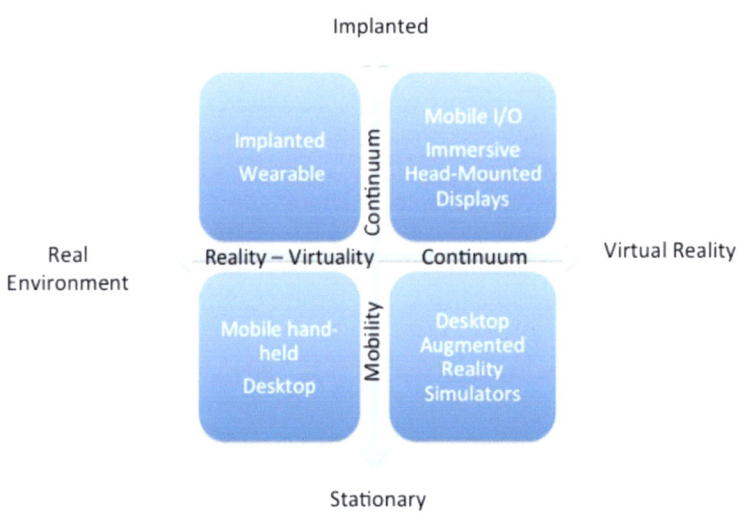

FIGURE 2-1 Range of options for cognitive artifacts.

Augmented Reality

One special category is augmented reality (AR), in which, for example, a head-mounted display (HMD), eyeglass display, or embedded display identifies the objects around a person and supplies valuable information. AR has become common: smart phones have this capability, and it is being built into automobiles, sometimes within a head-up display (HUD) for the driver. Military uses dominate in this arena; HUDs are common in aircraft or mounted on the visors of combat helmets.

There are two forms of AR: strong and weak. In strong AR, information is superimposed on the perceived world. In weak AR, information is available on auxiliary displays. In the commercial world, the distinction is best illustrated by the difference between wearing goggles, which superimpose the names of perceived buildings and objects over the objects themselves (strong AR), and using a smart phone, whereby a photograph of an object is interpreted and overlaid with the name of the object (weak AR). Although the information conveyed by strong and weak AR systems is often identical, the format of strong AR is faster and easier to perceive and use than that of weak AR.

In either strong or weak AR, perceptual information is augmented by computer-generated displays that annotate the visual information and amplify or otherwise enhance auditory or tactile information. In some cases, the sensory modality may become transformed so that information in one domain is perceivable in others. Light waves outside the visible spectrum might get false coloring to make them perceivable. Acoustic signals outside the range of hearing might be modified to lie within the normal frequency range. Sensory signals from the rear or side might be transformed into something within the sphere of attention (so that a vehicle outside the sphere might be represented by vibration on the back or relevant side), and electromagnetic spectra might get transformed into vibration, acoustic signals, or visible light.

There is a class of computational support that reduces human error, increases efficiency and throughput, and simultaneously avoids interference with command decisions or regulated (validated) software, such as some software found in the medical-device industry. Henry Lieberman defined agents for the user interface in his text with Ted Selker that describes a concept that he had introduced earlier: the advisor agent (Lieberman and Selker, 2003; Lieberman, 1998). Conceptually, the advisor agent provides digital support to human cognition—real-time management of complex, multidimensional, or dynamic issue tracking (for example, what not to forget in the process of going from state A to state B or alerts to what is changing in the background, how fast, and with what impact). Medtronic, Inc. described an advisor agent that has reduced error rate, increased throughput, and reduced costs by more than $ 300,000 per year in issue tracking and resolution for operating software in implantable medical devices (Drew and Gini, 2012; Drew and Goetz, 2008). The net effect has been to augment the cognitive capability of the software engineer by increasing precision and fidelity while reducing tedium.

Many of the ideas in this field are used in commercial applications, especially games and automobile safety systems. Military applications are obvious and are already being deployed.

Socially Distributed Augmented Reality

One important subject of research is socially distributed augmented cognition, whereby multiple people experience the same events and each is capable of contributing expertise. One of the presenters to this committee, Thad Starner, wore a head-mounted camera and display, a chord keyboard in his pocket, and a computer and communication system in his backpack. While in the committee meeting in Irvine, California, he was in continuous contact with his research group at Georgia Tech in Atlanta, Georgia. They were able to see what he was seeing, to hear the committee discussion, and to provide him with relevant information and literature sources in real time on his HMD. (Because of continual difficulties with the communication link, the demonstration did not always work—an illustration of both the strengths and the shortcomings of the current technology.)

This form of AR has great potential in command and decision modes, in which different external experts can provide relevant information and interpretation even while they are in remote and geographically dispersed locations.

Mobile augmented reality (MAR) extends the AR paradigm, which is to display digital information in the user's view via HMD or other display so that objects in the physical world and digital world appear to coexist spatially (Milgram and Kishino, 1994). Through the use of location-aware mobile devices, MAR can broaden the interaction space of traditional AR, in which the augmented interaction space is limited to a predefined area, and contribute to mobile learning that takes advantage of the context and manner in which people receive information with respect to their environment (Liu and Milrad, 2010).

An example of a MAR learning tool is ARCHEOGUIDE, which provides virtual reconstructions of artifacts and buildings and site-specific information about historic places in the real environment (Gleue and Dähne, 2001). In this early MAR system, users wore an HMD and a backpack full of sensors and mobile equipment. The concept was extended to games and tourist applications, including TimeWarp (Herbst, et al., 2008) and Science in the City AR (Roschelle, 2003). It has also been extended to create new forms of artistic expression—artworks not visible outside the MAR environment (http://www.unseensculptures.com).

In MAR systems, augmentable targets can be streets, buildings, natural areas and objects, and even people and other moving targets. MAR enables the physical environment to be directly annotated and described in situ, guiding users to pay attention to particular parts of objects in their environment. Virtually any object in the user's environment could become a point of entry to new information; that is, "the world becomes the user interface" and material for learning (Höllerer and Feiner, 2004; Welch and Bishop, 1997). This is a great opportunity to design new educational technologies that aim to connect learning materials to students' personal lives and experience beyond the classroom. In contrast with traditional educational materials, MAR systems can provide students with ways to connect classroom concepts more directly and interactively with examples found in the real environment.

In addition to its mobility, MAR is a unique enabler for mobile learning because of its multimodality and its ability to simulate new perspectives directly in the user's environment. Through visually rich simulations and location-sensitive media, MAR can provide people with new or alternative ways of looking at the world. For example, the see-through vision system of Avery et al. (2008) allowed visualization of occluded objects in an outdoor setting, textured with real-time video information. Their MAR system gave people access to a kind of "x-ray vision", revealing the activities that were taking place inside a building from outside. Similarly, an underground visualization system gave users 3-D models of the underground infrastructure superimposed on a construction site. The MARCH (Mobile Augmented Reality for Cultural Heritage) system was designed to help users to identify cave drawings by overlaying experts' drawings on top of the surface of the cave (Choudary et al., 2009). The Earthquake AR explored how MAR could be used to visualize reconstructed buildings and to show other earthquake-related information on site after a disaster (Billinghurst and Grasset, 2010). After the earthquake in Christchurch, New Zealand, people walked around the city with Earthquake AR and saw life-sized virtual models of buildings where the buildings themselves had been.

In summary, instead of immersing people in a virtual world, MAR enables people to remain connected with their physical environment and invites them to look at the world from new, alternative perspectives (Ryokai and Agogino, in press). By presenting alternative perspectives in their everyday view, MAR could facilitate a richer perception of the everyday environment.

Enhanced Cognitive Performance Through Better Human-Centered Design

One important form of enhancement should not be overlooked: the design of human-centered systems. Today, many systems are not designed to enhance human performance. On the contrary, they are designed with the technical components of the system in mind and with an assumption that the person will handle any difficulties that arise. One result is that opportunities for enhancement are missed. A worse result is a high percentage of system failures, often blamed on "human error."

A rich body of literature demonstrates that "human error" is often the result of poor design. Machines can execute precise, repetitive operations; people are poorly suited to these tasks. On the other hand, people can perform well where flexibility and creativity are involved, and can react to novel, unexpected situations, whereas machines do poorly in this regard. But instead of taking advantage of the human virtues in designing systems, we often force people to operate by machine rules and logic. The result is that most accidents (the percentage varies from 75 percent to 90 percent) are blamed on humans.

With better attention to the well-established principles of human-centered design and human-systems integration, including modeling and simulation of human cognitive performance, we could get huge enhancement in human cognitive capability with no need for new research or new applications. The principles are well known—they can be found in many books, courses, conferences, and tutorials. For example, the Army MANPRINT program tries to ensure that they are used. In the National Research Council, the Board on Human-Systems Integration has issued report after report on this problem (e.g., NRC, 1997a, 1997b, 2005, 2007, 2011). Donald A.

Norman's comments to the committee show how the past reports have been operationalized (Norman, 2011).

The United States has a competitive advantage in the development of human-centered software. However, Siemens AG, a German company, and Delmia, a French company, are the two major suppliers of advanced human simulation software in this arena. Other countries either do not pay as much attention to these issues or are still dominated by an engineering mentality that puts the needs of the machines first and the capabilities of people second. Moreover, Eastern cultures, which emphasize the needs of society over those of the individual, are at a disadvantage in this particular domain in that the individual must often learn to comply with societal demands. This philosophy seldom translates into human-centered software design.

Thoughts on the Concept of Radical Innovation in Cognitive Enhancement

A major concern for this committee is how radical innovation might suddenly appear and redefine cognitive enhancement. Although it is often believed that this is a result of detailed research and the invention of new technologies, that is not necessarily the case.

Two recent examples are pertinent of off-the-shelf technologies that were given amazing new uses:

- Siri, a spinoff venture of SRI International, which launched the product, was bought by Apple one month later and now is a major part of the iPhone.
- Nintendo Wii revolutionized the game industry by using existing technologies that had been ignored by competitors.

Siri integrates Nuance Corporation's speech-recognition system (and text-to-speech) with standard simple artificial intelligence and database techniques, thus leveraging many services that were already on the Web (such as Wolfram's Alpha and Wikipedia) in a software-as-a-service architecture. Wii introduced the use of infrared imaging chips and inexpensive sensors (spurned by other game-makers because they were thinking only of bigger and faster graphics and processing) and redefined the game industry. Microsoft Kinect can be considered a descendant of the Wii concept in that once Microsoft engineers understood the Wii architecture, they were able to put together elements that were already in their laboratories with a commercially available 3-D ranging camera. Both Wii and Kinect have been shown to have HPM applications: Wii has been used for integrated cognitive and physical therapy in assisted-living environments (Rolland et al., 2007), and Kinect has been used to integrate cognitive tasks with physical movement for improvements in learning (Lo, 2012).

History repeatedly illustrates that a lot of so-called revolutionary technology comes about simply through the reframing and redefining of an existing product. New technologies and scientific breakthroughs are not always required. That presents a challenge in identifying and tracking "radical" innovation: when it is simply the result of reimagining what can be done with existing components, little warning is available.

Cognitive Degradation

Every technology that is meant to enhance human performance can, under the wrong circumstances, reduce human performance. This degradation of performance may not be deliberate (e.g., cell phone texting while driving) or it may be deliberate. In an example of the latter, two Japanese researchers developed a delayed-speech feedback system (Kurihara and Tsukada, 2012). It uses the well-known phenomenon in speech whereby playing a speaker's voice back to the speaker with a delay of 0.2 - 0.3 seconds interferes with speech production; it can produce intense stuttering. The Japanese system uses commercial components: a directional microphone coupled with a highly directional loudspeaker to record and delay a voice and then beam it back to the speaking human. It is conceivable that this technique would work over considerable distances.

The committee did not find other examples of degradation, but it appears to be a potentially valuable subject that is so far largely unexplored. Obvious forms of degradation, including the distribution of false information (such as spoofing, counterfeiting, false trails, and false leaks) are well known and are standard in novels and movies. Other disruptions interfere with the communication channel, as in the example above—it is a form of "denial of service." This kind of attack is also well known. Nonetheless, the committee found little evidence of the use of technologies of cognitive enhancement for performance degradation.

Foreign Research in Cognitive Modification

The committee was unable to discover topics related to cognitive enhancement that were being pursued exclusively outside the United States. As in the United States, most such work is either being done in research laboratories and published openly or is being introduced into commercial products. Unpublished or classified work that cannot be discovered through normal channels might be occurring within the United States; and discovering such foreign work is even more difficult.

One of the committee's advisors on technologies for augmented cognition reported that funding for applications was difficult to get in the United States but that other countries had increased their support:

> . . . 2005 . . . was the year that Europe and Asia really started betting on ubicomp/wearables (ubiquitous computing and wearables). We are seeing the results now—Europe has been pulling ahead of U.S. steadily in wearables/ubicomp research, and South Korea is starting to surpass U.S. in electronic textiles research, in my opinion. Much of my wearables research and funding is with the EU and South Korea. My colleagues in China seem to be suddenly in demand for projects they can't talk about with me or their European friends (military?). Though China is behind U.S. in research, Foxconn has an internal start-up on Head Up Displays (HUDs)—they bought out much of the Myvu/MicroOptical management and patents after they closed. (Thad Starner, personnel communication, March 2012)

3
Human Performance Modification as a Biological Problem

Several technologies that can affect human biological systems are fertile ground for exploration of how human performance can be modified. These include tissue engineering, methods for combating fatigue related to the operational cycles of the human body, and issues associated with nutrition. Because nutrition was explicitly excluded from its task, the committee has restricted its discussion to human tissue engineering and fatigue research.

TISSUE ENGINEERING

The modification of the cellular aspects of humans is a subject of active inquiry throughout the world. The types of tissues that are being researched range from muscles (e.g., to increase strength) to organs (e.g., to create replacement organs). The research is being conducted in sports-medicine laboratories, genetic-engineering laboratories, and rehabilitative-surgery centers. The committee found tissue engineering to be one of the most difficult subjects to review because it is so vast, so varied, and so complex. Further, because the topic involves direct interference in the human body, there are widely differing views around the world as to what kinds of research are considered morally acceptable.

Tissue engineering can be defined as the use of cells, engineering, materials, and suitable biochemical and physiochemical factors to improve or replace biological functions. Success has been achieved in tissues that are thin membranes, that are avascular, or that have high regeneration potential. For example, tissue-engineered skin, cartilage, bone, and corneas have been used clinically (Khademhosseini et al., 2009).

There have been three approaches to tissue engineering: the conductive approach, using a material to provide the structural framework for cell infiltration; the inductive approach, using soluble materials to promote cell infiltration; and the cell-replacement approach, providing either an allograft (from a donor) or an autologous graft (from the patient) to repair a tissue. Those approaches have been successfully used clinically to improve regeneration. Tissue engineering can be used to speed recovery and to improve the quality of the generated tissue.

In the case of cell-replacement therapies, the cell source is of great importance. With a shortage of donor organs and available cells, stem cells are the primary alternative to isolating cells from a patient's tissue (Doss et al., 2004). Human embryonic stem cells, which have the capacity to differentiate into all cell types, have resulted in the formation of teratomas[1] when implanted in vivo (Thomson et al., 1998; Caspi et al., 2007). Adult stem cells, which can

---

[1] A teratoma is a "multi-layered benign tumor that grows from pluripotent cells injected into mice with a dysfunctional immune system. Scientists test whether they have established a human embryonic stem cell (hESC) line by injecting putative stem cells into such mice and verifying that the resulting teratomas contain cells derived from all three embryonic germ layers." National Institutes of Health, U.S. Department of Health and Human Services. 2011. Stem Cell Information. Available at http://stemcells.nih.gov/info/glossary. Accessed August 10, 2012.

differentiate into several but not all cell types, have been in use for decades. Hematopoietic[2] and mesenchymal[3] stem cells are commonly used but have limited capacity. Primary cells, or terminally differentiated cells, lack the capacity to regenerate numerous times, and often cell quality decreases with each passage.

Today, most tissues are too complex to be replicated. First, the ability to create a vascularized tissue remains a fundamental challenge in the field. Mass-transport limitations governing nutrients and waste affect the function and viability of a tissue (Allen et al., 2001; Sachlos and Auguste, 2008). Microfluidic, capillary-like systems exhibit high resistance and require substantial pressures to produce continuous flow. Second, the ability to organize cells in three dimensions is limited. Hydrogel-based and scaffold-based matrices offer little help in the assembly of cellular networks, which are important for cell–cell communication. For example, the heart and muscles must contract synchronously. Discontinuities within the cell organization can result in loss of function or abnormal gene expression, which can lead to a diseased state. Thus, cell organization, mechanics, and electric signals must all be linked to produce a viable, functional tissue.

Focused efforts have tried to repair tissue by mimicking 3-D tissue architecture, extracellular matrix, and cell organization. For example, organ printing was established as a bottom-up approach that uses 100- to 500-μm aggregates of cells, known as tissue spheroids, as building blocks to make 3-D tissue constructs (Ruei-Zeng and Hwan-You, 2008). Robotic bioprinting of hydrogel droplets containing cells can be used to dispense or digitally spray tissue spheroids to achieve multicellular structures (Wang et al., 2006). Cells then self-assemble within and between spheroids to form larger, integrated structures. However, mass-transport limitations hinder the advancement of this technology.

In summary, the ability to enhance tissue performance is limited by (1) the need to obtain adequate and substantial numbers of viable cells, (2) mass-transport characteristics that dictate cell viability, and (3) the need to recapitulate the tissue architecture and cell organization that are required for tissue function. Tissue-engineering methods are focused on clinical repair, and current methods are unable to surpass the functioning of healthy tissue.

Worldwide Research

Tissue engineering has commercial applications in ligament repair and replacement, and epidermal constructs. The committee found that the countries with companies that provide products in this field include Australia, France, Italy, Germany, the United States, the United Kingdom, Switzerland, Japan, and Korea. Research on organ regeneration and bone replacement is also under way.

FATIGUE: JUDGMENT AND DECISION MAKING

Good human–machine system design exploits human strengths (such as pattern recognition and decision making) and protects against human weaknesses. "The human operator brings much more performance variability to a system than one finds in [reliable] software and modern hardware. . . . Once an operator has been trained and is current in system operation, the greatest

---

[2] "Hematopoietic stem cells are immature cells that develop into all types of blood cells including white blood cells, red blood cells and platelets." National Institutes of Health, U.S. Department of Health and Human Services. 2011. Stem Cell Information. Available at http://stemcells.nih.gov/info/glossary. Accessed July 31, 212. For more information on hematopoietic stem cells, see http://stemcells.nih.gov/info/basics/basics4.asp. Accessed July 31, 2012.

[3] Mesenchymal stem cells are "rare cells mainly found in the bone marrow that can give rise to a large number of tissue types such as bone, cartilage (the lining of joints), fat tissue and connective tissue (tissue that is in between organs and structures in the body)." Texas Heart Institute. 2009. Available at http://texasheart.org/Research/StemCellCenter/Glossary.cfm. Accessed July 31, 2012.

contributor to variability in that person's performance is cognitive fatigue," especially during night work (Folkard and Tucker, 2003; Miller 2005, 2010).

The human body has complex operational requirements, one of which is adequate rest. During rest periods, such as sleep, vital functions occur (Matthews et al., 2012). When the body is deprived of rest, specifically sleep, those functions do not occur, and the ability of the person to perform degrades predictably. The effect is noticeable in both cognitive and muscular performance. Sleep deprivation also causes substantial physiologic changes, such as increases in blood pressure (Conquest, 1991; Matthews et al., 2012; Chan et al., 1993).

The need for sleep is complicated by the reaction of the human body to light and dark. Sleep during periods of light is not as effective in operational restoration of the human mechanism as sleep during periods of darkness. Research has shown that job effectiveness, as measured in terms of the speed and accuracy of trained workers, is highest between 7 a.m. and 7 p.m. and lowest during the predawn hours (Fokard and Tucker, 2003; Office of Technology Assessment, 1991).

Physical fatigue in people is manifested in deteriorated dexterity, decreased eye–hand coordination, tremors, discomfort, and loss of strength and endurance. It is often not only how long a person works or how much rest and sleep he or she receives, but also the type of physical and mental workload that the person is subjected to while awake that determines whether fatigue is present (Chaffin et al., 2006).

System design can play an important part in improving or optimizing the performance of human elements in the overall system (Costa, 2001). Conversely, human performance can be degraded by taking advantage of perturbations to normal operational cycles (for example, attacking before dawn) (Gunzelman et al., 2012).

Some research in the various aspects of human fatigue is focusing on how human performance can be modified—improved or degraded—through fatigue-related elements of system design and performance (Matthews et al., 2012). Research tends to be focused on working situations in which altered sleep patterns are necessary, such as military movements or shift-work environments (Hull, 1990; Office of Technology Assessment, 1991; West et al., 2007; Samaha et al., 2007).

It is clear that fatigue-inducing situations degrade human performance. They can lead to dangerous situations, such as when a transport worker's decision-making ability is degraded because of fatigue. Research has shown that fatigue has serious effects on the human brain (Reeves et al., 2006, 2007). But research results are mixed as to how to optimize human sleep needs in operational environments that demand 24-hour activity, such as in medical facilities, prisons, manufacturing plants, and telecommunications facilities (Costa, 2001). The optimization of length and staggering of shift assignments are being studied, but no clear picture of a "right" answer has emerged. Each environment has a different type of worker and different operational requirements, and this may explain why the research findings are mixed.

Some technologies can affect fatigue. For example, there has been a revolution in the science and technology of light-induced human performance modification. The use of spectrum-tuned light sources can wake people up or cause them to become drowsy. Examples are the recent identification of the melanopsin-pigmented retinal ganglion cell system, which is exquisitely sensitive to 460- to 480-nm blue light, and the use of blue-light filtering (in Canada) and blue-light treatment (in Europe) to affect human performance in 24/7 operations. The energy in that narrow window—6 percent of the total visual light spectrum—can duplicate the effects of the energy of the total light spectrum. These developments can be expected to influence the design of lighting systems, computer display screens, and eyewear. For example, Casper (at the University of Toronto) has shown that filtering out 460- to 480-nm light dramatically improves vigilance and performance in the circadian nadir (Rahman et al., 2011); it reverses the nocturnal dip in performance and provides users an enormous advantage in nighttime and early-morning operations.

The practical applications of such technologies are being explored in various situations, such as military deployments and long-haul trucking (Paul et al., 2007). Paul and his Canadian colleagues have successfully countered jet lag and shift lag by timing light treatments in conjunction with timing ingestion of sustained-release melatonin. Light treatments are also being used in the treatment of seasonal affective disorder. The physiologic mechanisms are still being explored (Boivin and James, 2005; James et al., 2004). A combination of the technologies with pharmacologic agents, such as caffeine or melatonin, and structured changes in sleep patterns can assist people who must move between time zones (Piérard et al., 2001).

Most fatigue researchers point out that the solutions to worker fatigue include the participation of workers' organizations, managers, and supervisors. Fatigue is difficult for people to manage successfully apart from their work environments. Enormous strides have been made in the design, development, and implementation of fatigue-risk management systems (FRMSs). Regulations and laws have been passed that require FRMSs, as discussed in the comprehensive FRMS guidance statement published by the American College of Occupational and Environmental Medicine (Lerman et al., 2012).

Interestingly, some people are naturally fatigue-resistant (Aeschbach et al., 2003; He et al., 2009; King et al., 2009). There might be an identifiable genetic component of that attribute that has not yet been discovered. If such a genetic component is identified, it might be a useful target for experimentation to help workers or soldiers to become fatigue-resistant.

Knowledge about the nature of fatigue associated with many kinds of specific jobs may be used to optimize operational plans. International working-time regulations may affect military or contractor duty periods during training. The accident and incident risks associated with fatigue may be documented and quantified, and the results may inform operational planning. In the next 5 years, 12-hour shifts may come to dominate 24/7 operations because of the flexibility they provide workers to structure their off-duty time. Technologies for ambient light treatment in the nighttime workplace have been deployed commercially and may be used to enhance nighttime work performance. Readiness-for-duty testing technologies have been deployed minimally in the commercial world (Axelsson et al., 1998; Bloodworth et al., 2001; Campolo et al., 1998; Dwyer et al., 2007; Laundry and Lees, 1991; McGettrick and O'Neill, 2006; Richardson et al., 2007; Smith et al., 1998; Tucker et al., 1998; Williamson et al., 1994).

In the next 5-10 years, fatigue-risk modeling will become common in 24/7 operations. Modafinil may be approved as an over-the-counter stimulant to be used somewhat like caffeine. Top-down FRMSs will be common in 24/7 operations, and the practice of removing sleep debt before critical operations will also be common. In the next 10-15 years, pretravel adjustment of the circadian rhythm will become common, and on-duty napping during 24/7 and nighttime operations will become an accepted practice. In the next 15-20 years, rapidly rotating and flexible shift plans will be used in support of 24/7 operations, and more care will be taken to ensure that enough personnel will be available to support four- and five-crew solutions to meet 24/7 work demand (Axelsson et al., 1998; Bloodworth et al., 2001; Campolo et al., 1998; Dwyer et al., 2007; Laundry and Lees, 1991; McGettrick and O'Neill, 2006; Richardson et al., 2007; Smith et al., 1998; Tucker et al., 1998; Williamson et al., 1994).

There are some indications that physiological stimulation of the human body can interfere with sleep biology (De Groen, 1979). At the crudest level, such stimulation might be a physical nudge. At the most sophisticated level, it might be brain stimulation (Dimitrov and Ralev, 2009). It is well within the realm of imagination to consider the potential of implants, such as electrodes, that might provide such stimulation if a series of warning indicators were detected. Alerts based on measurement of ocular movements and blinks have been used successfully to reduce impairment caused by drowsiness in real time in equipment-operating tasks (Johns et al., 2007).[4]

---

[4]Fletcher, Adam. 2012. "Technologies for Fatigue Detection and Management." Presentation to the committee, March 8.

The alerts have been effective temporarily, but additional research is needed to assess their full impact on fatigue. Recent advances in integration of computing power into personally wearable devices, such as smart wristwatches, will probably contribute to advances in the ability to measure and respond to physiologic changes that indicate fatigue.

Worldwide Research

The committee found that open research in human fatigue is being conducted in several countries: Belgium, Australia, the Netherlands, Germany, Canada, Japan, the United Kingdom, the United States, Kuwait, Italy, France, Poland, and Singapore.

4
Human Performance Modification as a Function of Brain–Computer Interfaces

BRAIN–COMPUTER INTERFACES

This chapter reviews recent progress in brain-computer interfaces (BCIs), including the potentially enabling role of nanotechnology. BCIs allow direct communication of neural signals with an external device. A large body of research concerns the ability to detect and translate neural activity, direct it to control a machine, and thereby affect human performance (Brunner et al., 2011). The most common applications are in rehabilitative medicine. For example, neural implants now enable a disabled patient to control a wheelchair, prosthesis, or voice simulator (Rebsamen et al., 2010; Bell et al., 2008; Brumberg and Guenther, 2010). Conversely, electronic signals may be used to stimulate portions of the brain to induce a particular motor response; this has been demonstrated only in animals (Arfin et al., 2009; Nuyujukian et al., 2011). All of the BCIs in current use appear to be very slow and do not perform as well as a healthy person can.

Detection of Electric Signals

Several elements are required for a BCI to work. Perhaps the most important is that the brain signals are detected and understood. When a neuron fires, it emits a detectable electric signal. That is most commonly detected externally and noninvasively by electroencephalography (EEG), in which electrodes are placed on the scalp. EEG is widely used for detection of electrical activity associated with epileptic seizures or to characterize the overall status of electrical activity in the brain (Wolpaw et al., 2002). Researchers have made much progress in understanding which regions of the brain are activated during particular processes. Recent studies at the University of California, Berkeley have shown that it is possible to reconstruct sounds heard by a patient suffering from severe epilepsy on the basis of EEG spectra obtained from neural probes implanted in his brain (Pasley et al., 2012). The next step would be to extend the capability to analyze EEG spectra of thoughts and convert them to speech. This would be an exciting advance, in that it could allow people who have lost the ability to speak to recover it.

In the military realm, fighter-pilot helmets lined with EEG sensors have been developed as part of a cognitive avionics tool set (Schnell, 2009). The goal is to collect as much data as possible to measure pilot cognitive overloading and underloading in high-stress situations. However, the most important indicators of these conditions to date are eye-gaze and respiration data rather than EEG data. To make EEG data more useful, synchronization systems that can correlate EEG response to pilot expertise need to be developed. Research is continuing to extract higher-resolution and more useful information from the EEG data by using higher frequencies for better topographic resolution and by creating much denser arrays of electrodes; the latter is now possible with soft materials and advanced fabrication methods (Crone et al., 2006).

In addition to detecting brain activity externally, it is possible to implant devices directly into the brain. The advantage is that the electrodes are much closer to the source of electrical activity, so the signal-to-noise ratio is greatly improved and the localization provides a more direct idea of the origin of the activity (Vetter et al., 2003). A number of such devices have been developed (primarily in the United States), notably BRAINGATE, the Utah Probe, and the Michigan Probe (Archibald, 2005; Huys et al., 2011; Kipke et al., 2011). Such invasive probes or arrays of an EEG type of electrodes on the surface of the brain are contemplated only for patients who have severe disorders. The smallest probes currently available are much larger than individual neurons; serious damage is done to brain tissue on insertion, and the process is irreversible (He et al., 2006). It may be justified for severely disabled patients, but seems unlikely to be acceptable as an enhancement method in the near term. Major efforts are under way in a number of laboratories to integrate electrodes or meshes of electrodes with neurons (and other cell types) in culture, and this is potentially a less destructive approach (Lee et al., 2004). It has potential for repair of damaged neuronal tissue, including the possibility of using radiofrequency electronics so that signals can be read—or regions can be stimulated—remotely.

Functional Detection

An alternative detection system is related more directly to physiology, particularly blood flow and glucose metabolism associated with activity in a particular region of the brain (Son and Yazici, 2005). That is the basis of functional magnetic resonance imaging (fMRI), positron-emission tomography (PET), and near-infrared functional (NIRF) imaging. Although fMRI and PET imaging are major imaging modalities in clinical medicine and brain research, neither can currently be implemented in a portable or even semiportable format (Son and Yazici, 2005).

NIRF imaging uses changes in the near-infrared absorption of deoxyhemoglobin vs. oxyhemoglobin to obtain information on changes in blood oxygenation (Cui et al., 2011; Hoshi, 2011). Blood oxygenation changes during high levels of activity, and substantial changes are observed in brain tissue. Arrays of near-infrared sources (for example, laser diodes) and detectors in combination can be used to generate low-resolution images of brain function. The penetration of near-infrared light through the skull of adults is modest (it is much higher in premature infants, and this technique is used in the neonatal intensive care unit).

Using brain signals to monitor cognition for use in training has demonstrated benefits. Some groups are pursuing augmented cognition whereby human performance is improved by designing for memorability. It is necessary for cognitive bottlenecks and firing patterns to be measured to detect cognitive states within some small amount of time (Son and Yazici, 2005). If that can be accomplished, perhaps behavior can be influenced.

Although a great deal of progress has been made in this realm, how the brain functions is still largely unknown (Son and Yazici, 2005; Hoshi, 2011). Even if neural events could be reliably correlated to the detection of sensory inputs or to the stimulation of specific motor activity, there is a fundamental issue of neuromuscular mismatch (Kirilina et al., 2012). The brain has evolved to control muscles, whereas BCI research strives to create interfaces between the brain and computers. Current neural implants are rather crude, and a more biological way to create an interface with the brain to enhance efficacy and decrease scarring is being sought and may be found in the next 20 years. The most promising direct applications of this research to human performance modification (HPM) are in developing therapies for existing disabilities. Even in those cases, the improvements do not approach the functionality of a healthy person. It is unlikely that human performance can be substantially enhanced via BCI in the near term.

Worldwide Research

According to Thomas Schnell of the University of Iowa, non-U.S. entities appear to be more active in such cognitive-function research. He believes that the international players that warrant attention are Israel, Germany, Japan, and the Netherlands. It should also be noted that Taiwan and South Korea have infrastructure and expertise in these fields; for example, the Korea Advanced Institute of Science and Technology has recently established a Department of Bio and Brain Engineering. There is also great interest in this research in China. The work that has been published in western peer-reviewed scientific journals suggests that China is still building expertise based on western innovation rather than pioneering novel research of its own. Nonetheless, China is pouring resources into this area.[1]

Other Kinds of Interfaces

In the context of HPM, it is important to consider possibilities beyond physical modification of the human or the human's work environment. An intriguing example is that it may be possible to train a person to work with a machine or computer interface to enhance the person's normal capabilities (Cui et al., 2012). A crude illustration of this concept can be seen in the case of a bicycle. A person is trained to create an interface with the bicycle to increase his or her ability to move. The person learns to move his or her legs in a specific way to move the pedals to produce propulsion, to balance his or her body on the machine, and to maneuver the machine through combinations of body movements and steering. A more advanced illustration might be the training of a person to manipulate machines through the coordinated movements and controlled thought patterns that are accessible with increasingly sensitive equipment. The concept would build on capabilities that are already in place, such as eye-movement measurements and body-tracking capabilities. An example of a nascent capability of this kind can be seen in the University of Washington application[2] that uses a kinesthetic learning environment to teach students mathematics. The idea of training the user and the machine together may open a new frontier in HPM. Augmenting performance may not require as much if machine and user are trained together as it would otherwise.

NANOTECHNOLOGY FOR HUMAN PERFORMANCE MODIFICATION

Nanotechnology involves any application of materials that measure a few hundreds of nanometers or smaller. It can refer to a wide variety of technologies relevant to HPM, including electronics, microelectromechanical systems, energy harvesting and storage, and biomedicine. The field cuts across many of the other aspects of HPM in that it enables their implementation.

Advanced fabrication techniques allow ever-smaller computer chips, cameras, and antennae that can result in wireless devices that are small and light enough to be integrated into virtually every aspect of human endeavor. Smart phones, for instance, benefit from these advances, allowing more capabilities to be integrated in a device that is small and light enough to fit in a pocket. Devices such as smart phones arguably enhance human performance by making a vast amount of information accessible. The miniaturization is also enabling technologies that more directly alter human performance, such as proposed wearable augmented reality devices, including Sixth Sense—an interface based on gestures that is a predecessor of the type depicted in

---

[1]Thomas Schnell, Associate Professor, University of Iowa. Operator State Characterization Using Neurophysiological Measures. Presentation to the committee on March 8, 2012.

[2]For more information, see http://kinectmath.org/. Accessed August 2, 2012.

the film *Minority Report*—and Google Glasses, a heads-up display that promises to project smartphone functionality in the wearer's field of view.[3,4]

Another aspect of nanotechnology that needs to be considered with regard to HPM is in the realm of biointerfaces. Nanoparticles can be smaller than cells, and this opens the possibility of using them to interact directly on a cellular level by inserting them into the body. A straightforward application is to enhance sensory perception via subdermal nanoparticles. Recently, Nokia filed a patent for a tattoo containing nanoparticles that vibrate when a cell-phone call is received.[5] It is easy to imagine how such a consumer device can be applied to the battlefield; for instance, the tattoo could be coupled to chemical sensors to alert soldiers to the presence of toxic gases or explosives.

A more invasive use of nanotechnology for HPM is in the development of neural implants. These devices are implanted directly into the brain to detect electric signaling. To increase the signal-to-noise ratio and resolution, the probes need to be on the same scale as the neurons that they monitor, that is, a few micrometers. Furthermore, they must be made of materials that are biocompatible and produce little or no damage and scarring of the surrounding tissue. To achieve that, sophisticated nanomaterials are being developed.

Worldwide Research

Although much of the research in nanotechnology began in the United States, continued development for electronics and related applications is taking place globally, spurred largely by the consumer and military markets. U.S. superiority in the development of these and newer technologies cannot be assumed, especially given that a large fraction of the manufacturing of state-of-the-art electronics is taking place in Asia. The United States is a leader in basic research in neural engineering, but laboratories in Europe and in Asia (China in particular) are also active.

---

[3]For more information about Sixth Sense, see http://www.pranavmistry.com/projects/sixthsense. Accessed May 3, 2012.

[4]For more information about Google Glasses, see https://plus.google.com/u/0/111626127367496192147/posts. Accessed May 3, 2012.

[5]For more information, see https://docs.google.com/file/d/0B23n8sehUZyqckhLaG9qZ0hRSXFnQkctYXhDYTY4dw/edit?pli=1. Accessed June 27, 2012.

Bibliography

Aeschbach, D., L. Sher, T.T. Postolache, J.R. Matthews, M.A. Jackson, and T.A. Wehr. 2003. A longer biological night in long sleepers than in short sleepers. Journal of Clinical Endocrinology and Metabolism 88(1):26-30.

Agogino, A.M., and R. Payo. 2007. "K-12 Resources in the NSDL Engineering Pathway," presentation at the workshop entitled "The Power of Digital Libraries: Inquiry-Based and Experiential Learning and Teaching," AAAS Annual Meeting, February 16, San Francisco, Calif. Available at http://www.pr2ove-it.org/shared/publications/AAAS_k-12.htm.

Agogino, A.M., and B. Muramatsu. 1997. The National Engineering Education Delivery System (NEEDS): A multimedia digital library of courseware. International Journal of Engineering Education 13(5):333-340.

Al-Kahtani, N., J.C.H. Ryan, and T.I. Jefferson. 2005/2006. How Saudi female faculty perceive internet technology usage and potential. Information Knowledge Systems Management 5(4):227-243.

Albrecht, R., T. Lokki, and L. Savioja. 2011. A mobile augmented reality audio system with binaural microphones. Pp. 7-11 in Proceedings of Interacting with Sound Workshop: Exploring Context-Aware, Local and Social Audio Applications. New York, N.Y.: Association for Computing Machinery.

Allen, C.B., B.K. Schneider, and C.W. White. 2001. Limitations to oxygen diffusion and equilibration in in vitro cell exposure systems in hyperoxia and hypoxia. American Journal of Physiology-Lung Cellular and Molecular Physiology 281:L1021-L1027.

American Association for the Advancement of Science (AAAS). 2006. Human Enhancement and the Means of Achieving It. Washington, D.C.: AAAS. Available at http://www.aaas.org/spp/sfrl/projects/human_enhancement/achievingHEindex.shtml. Accessed June 21, 2012.

Amish Heartland. 2012. FAQ About the Amish. Available at http://www.amish-heartland.com/. Accessed June 21, 2012.

Archibald, S. 2005. Opening the BrainGate. Nature Review Neuroscience 6:346-346.

Arfin, S.K., M.A. Long, M.S. Fee, and R. Sarpeshkar. 2009. Wireless neural stimulation in freely behaving small animals. Journal of Neurophysiology 102:598-605.

Avery, B., B.H. Thomas, and W. Piekarski. 2008. User evaluation of see-through vision for mobile outdoor augmented reality. Pp. 69-72 in Proceedings of the 7th IEEE/ACM International Symposium on Mixed and Augmented Reality (ISMAR '08). Washington, D.C.: IEEE Computer Society.

Axelsson, J., G. Kecklund, T. Akerstedt, and A. Lowden. 1998. Effects of alternating 8- and 12-hour shifts on sleep, sleepiness, physical effort and performance. Scandinavian Journal of Work, Environment and Health 24(Suppl 3):62-68.

Azuma, R.T. 1993. Tracking requirements for augmented reality. Communications of the ACM 36(7):50-51.

Backus, J. 1978. Can programming be liberated from the von Neumann style? A functional style and its algebra of programs. Communications of the ACM 21:613. Available at http://www.cs.cmu.edu/~crary/819-f09/Backus78.pdf.

Bell, C.J., P. Shenoy, R. Chalodhorn, and R.P.N. Rao. 2008. Control of a humanoid robot by a noninvasive brain-computer interface in humans. Journal of Neural Engineering 5:214-220.

Benford, S., M. Flintham, A. Drozd, R. Anastasi, D. Rowland, N. Tandavanitj, M. Adams, J. Row-Farr, A. Oldroyd, and J. Sutton. 2004. Uncle Roy all around you: Implicating the city in a location-based performance. Proceedings of the International Conference on Advances in Computer Entertainment (ACE 2004).

Betzig, E., J.K. Trautman, T.D. Harris, R. Wolfe, E.M. Gregory, P.L. Finn, M.H. Kryder, and C.-H. Chang. 1992. Near-field magneto-optics and high density data storage. Applied Physics Letters 61:142

Billinghurst, M., H. Kato, and I. Poupyrev. 2001. The magicbook—Moving seamlessly between reality and virtuality. IEEE Computer Graphics and Applications 21(3):6-8.

Billinghurst, M., and R. Grasset. 2011. Earthquake AR. Available at http://www.hitlabnz.org/index.php/research/augmented-reality?view=project&task=show&id=24. Accessed June 29, 2012.

Blevis, E. 2007. Sustainable interaction design: Invention and disposal, renewal and reuse. Pp. 503-512 in Proceedings of the SIGCHI Conference on Human Factors in Computing Systems.

Bloodworth, C., A. Lea, S. Lane, and R. Ginn. 2001. Challenging the myth of the 12-hour shift: A pilot evaluation. Nursing Standard (Royal College of Nursing (Great Britain) 1987) 15(29):33-36.

Bobrich, J., and S. Otto. 2002. Augmented maps. In Geospatial Theory, Processing and Applications. Proceedings of ISPRS Commission IV, WG7. University of Hanover, Germany, Institute for Cartography and Geoinformatics.

Bohn, R., and J. Short, 2010. How Much Information? 2009: Report on American Consumers. University of California, San Diego: Global Information Industry Center.

Boivin, D.B., and F.O. James. 2005. Light treatment and circadian adaptation to shift work. Industrial Health 43(1):34-48.

Brown, J.S., A. Collins, and P. Duguid. 1989. Situated cognition and the culture of learning. Educational Researcher 18(1):32-42.

Brumberg, J.S., and F.H. Guenther. 2010. Development of speech prostheses: Current status and recent advances. Expert Review of Medical Devices 7:667-679.

Brunner, P., L. Bianchi, C. Guger, F. Cincotti, and G. Schalk. 2011. Current trends in hardware and software for brain-computer interfaces (BCIs). Journal of Neural Engineering 8:025001.

Campolo, M., J. Pugh, L. Thompson, and M. Wallace. 1998. Pioneering the 12-hour shift in Australia—Implementation and limitations. Australian Critical Care: Official Journal of the Confederation of Australian Critical Care Nurses 11(4):112-115.

Cash, K.J., and H.A. Clark. 2010. Nanosensors and nanomaterials for monitoring glucose in diabetes. Trends in Molecular Medicine 16(12):584-593.

Caspi, O., I. Huber, I. Kehat, M. Habib, G. Arbel, A. Gepstein, L. Yankelson, D. Aronson, R. Beyar, and L. Gepstein. 2007. Transplantation of human embryonic stem cell-derived cardiomyocytes improves myocardial performance in infarcted rat hearts. Journal of the American College of Cardiology 50:1884-1893.

Castle, R.O., G. Klein, and D.W. Murray. 2008. Video-rate localization in multiple maps for wearable augmented reality. Proceedings of 12th IEEE International Symposium on Wearable Computers, Pittsburgh, Pa., September 28-October 1.

Chaffin, D.B., G.B.J. Andersson, and B.J. Martin. 2006. Occupational Biomechanics. New York, N.Y.: John Wiley and Sons.

Chan, O., S. Gan, and M. Yeo. 1993. Study on the health of female electronics workers on 12 hour shifts. Occupational Medicine (Oxford, England) 43(3):143-148.

Cheok, A.D., K.H. Goh, W. Liu, F. Farbiz, S.W. Fong, S.L. Teo, Y. Li, and X. Yang. 2004. Human Pacman: A mobile, wide-area entertainment system based on physical, social, and ubiquitous computing. Personal and Ubiquitous Computing 8(2):71-81.

Choudary, O., V. Charvillat, R. Grigoras, and P. Gurdjos. 2009. MARCH: Mobile augmented reality for cultural heritage. Pp. 1023-1024 in Proceedings of the 17th ACM International Conference on Multimedia (MM '09). University of Toulouse, France. ACM, New York, N.Y.

Chua, L.O., and S.M. Kang. 1976. Memristive devices and systems. Proceedings of IEEE 64:209.

Clark, N., J. Blome, M. Chu, S. Mahlke, S. Biles, and K. Flautner. 2005. An architecture framework for transparent instruction set customization in embedded processors. Pp. 272-283 in Proceedings of the 32nd Annual International Symposium on Computer Architecture. doi:10.1109/ISCA.2005.9.

Conquest, R. 1991. The Great Terror. Oxford University Press, U.S.

Costa, G. 2001. The 24-hour society: Between myth and reality. Journal of Human Ergology 30(1-2):15-20.

Costabile, M.F., A. De Angeli, R. Lanzilotti, C. Ardito, P. Buono, and T. Pederson. 2008. Explore! Possibilities and challenges of mobile learning. Pp. 145-154 in Proceedings of CHI 2008. New York: ACM Press.

Crone, N.E., A. Sinai, and A. Korzeniewska. 2006. High-frequency gamma oscillations and human brain mapping with electrocorticography. Progress in Brain Research 159:275-295.

Crosby, P. 2012. The Square Kilometre Array. Industry Engagement Strategy 2012. Available at http://www.skatelescope.org/wp-content/uploads/2011/03/SKA-IES-ver-3-0.pdf

Csikszentmihalyi, M., and E. Rochberg-Halton. 1981. The Meaning of Things: Domestic Symbols and the Self. Cambridge University Press.

Cui, X., S. Bray, D.M. Bryant, G.H. Glover, and A.L. Reiss. 2011. A quantitative comparison of NIRS and fMRI across multiple cognitive tasks. Neuroimage 54:2808-2821.

Cui, X., D.M Bryant, and A.L. Reiss. 2012. NIRS-based hyperscanning reveals increased interpersonal coherence in superior frontal cortex during cooperation. Neuroimage 59:2430-2437.

CyberTracker. 2005. New Zealand. Available at http://www.cybertracker.co.za/.

De Groen, J.H. 1979. Influence of diffuse brain stimulation (DBS) on human sleep. I. Sleep pattern changes. Electroencephalography and Clinical Neurophysiology 46(6):689-695.

Dennard, R., F.H. Gaensslen, Y. Hwa-Nien, V.L. Rideout, E. Bassous, and A.R. Leblanc. 1974. Design of ion-implanted MOSFETs with very small physical dimensions. IEEE Journal of Solid State Circuits vSC-9:256. Available at http://www.ece.ucsb.edu/courses/ECE225/225_W07Banerjee/reference/Dennard.pdf. Accessed September 19, 2012.

Dewey, J., 1934. Art as Experience. Perigee Books.

Dimitrov, D.T., and N.D. Ralev. 2009. Signals and systems for electrosleep. Electronics and Electrical Engineering 5(93):95-98.

Doss, M.X., C.I. Koehler, C. Gissel, J. Hescheler, and A. Sachinidis. 2004. Embryonic stem cells: A promising tool for cell replacement therapy. Journal of Cellular and Molecular Medicine 8:465-473.

Drew, T., and M. Gini. 2012. Deployed: Advisor agent support for issue tracking in medical device development. In Proceedings of Twenty-Sixth AAAI Conference on Artificial Intelligence (AAAI-12), Twenty-Fourth Conference on Innovative Applications of Artificial Intelligence, Toronto, Canada, July 2012.

Drew, T., and S. Goetz. 2008. Vision of the virtual programmer—Steps towards change in instrument systems for implantable medical devices. Pp. 156-159 in Proceedings of the International Conference on Biomedical Electronics and Devices, Volume 1.

Dwyer, T., L. Jamieson, L. Moxham, D. Austen, and K. Smith. 2007. Evaluation of the 12-hour shift trial in a regional intensive care unit. Journal of Nursing Management 15(7):711-720. doi:10.1111/j.1365-2934.2006.00737.x.

Farabet, C., B. Martini, B. Corda, P. Akselrod, E. Culurciello, and Y. Lecun. 2011. NeuFlow: A runtime reconfigurable dataflow processor for vision. IEEE Computer Society Conference on Computer Vision and Pattern Recognition Workshops, 109.

Farabet, C., C. Poulet, Y. LeCun. 2009. An FPGA-based stream processor for embedded real-time vision with convolutional networks. IEEE 12th International Conference on Computer Vision, 879.

Ferrucci, D.A. 2012. Introduction to "This is Watson." IBM Journal of Research and Development 56(1):1.

Folkard, S., and P. Tucker. 2003. Shift work, safety and productivity. Occupational Medicine (Oxford, England) 53(2):95-101.

Freitas, R.A. 1996. Respirocytes—A Mechanical Artificial Red Cell: Exploratory Design in Medical Nanotechnology. Available at http://www.foresight.org/Nanomedicine/Respirocytes.html. Accessed June 21, 2012.

Gerber, B.L., A.M.L. Cavallo, and E.A. Marek. 2001. Relationships among informal learning environments, teaching procedures and scientific reasoning ability. International Journal of Science Education 23(5):535-549.

Ghani, A., T.M. McGinnity, L.P.Maguire, and J. Harkin, 2006. Area efficient architecture for large scale implementation of biologically plausible spiking neural networks on reconfigurable hardware. P. 939 in Proceedings of the International Conference on Field Programmable Logic and Applications.

Glackin, B., T.M. McGinnity, L.P. Maguire, Q.X. Wu, and A. Belatreche. 2005. Novel approach for the implementation of large-scale spiking neural networks on FPGAs. P. 552 in Proceedings of the Artificial Neural Network Conference.

Gleue, T., and P. Dähne. 2001. Design and implementation of a mobile device for outdoor augmented reality in the ARCHEOGUIDE project. Pp. 161-168 in Proceedings of the 2001 Conference on Virtual Reality, Archeology, and Cultural Heritage, Glyfada, Greece. ACM Press, New York, N.Y., and Computer Graphics Center, Darmstadt, Germany.

Goodwin, C. 1994. Professional vision. American Anthropologist 96(3):606-633.

Gschwind, M. 2007. The cell broadband engine: Exploiting multiple levels of parallelism in a chip multiprocessor. International Journal of Parallel Programming 35(3):233-262.

Gunzelman, G., K.A. Gluck, R.L. Moore, and D.F. Dinges. 2012. Diminished access to declarative knowledge with sleep deprivation. Cognitive Systems Research 13:1-11.

Hamann, H.F., Y.C. Martin, and H.K Wickramasinghe. 2004. Thermally-assisted recording beyond traditional limits. Applied Physics Letters 84:810.

Harkin, J., F. Morgan, S. Cawley, B. McGinley, S. Pande, U. McDaid, B. Glackin, and J. Maher. 2009. Exploring the evolution of NoC-based spiking neural networks on FPGAs. P. 300 in International Conference on Field Programmable Technology. Available at http://postgrad.ucc.ie/en/eedsp/Research/Papers/FMorganPapers/FMorganIEEE/F-MorganIEEE.pdf. Accessed September 19, 2012.

Hartenstein, R. 1997. The microprocessor is no more general purpose: Why future reconfigurable platforms will win. In Proceedings of the International Conference on Innovative Systems in Silicon, October 8-10, 1997, Austin, Tex.

He, Y., C.R. Jones, N. Fujiki, Y. Xu, B. Guo, J.L. Holder, M.J. Rossner, et al. 2009. The transcriptional repressor DEC2 regulates sleep length in mammals. Science 325(5942):866-870, doi:10.1126/science.1174443.

He, W., G.C. McConnell, and R.V. Bellamkonda. 2006. Nanoscale laminin coating modulates cortical scarring response around implanted silicon microelectrode arrays. Journal of Neural Engineering 3:316-326.

Heinrich, M., B.H. Thomas, and S. Mueller. 2008. ARWeather: An augmented reality weather system. In Proceedings of the 7th IEEE/ACM International Symposium on Mixed and Augmented Reality (ISMAR '08). Washington, D.C.: IEEE Computer Society.

Herbst, I., A.-K. Braun, R. McCall, and W. Broll. 2008. TimeWarp: interactive time travel with a mobile mixed reality game. In Proceedings of MobileHCI 2008, September 2-5, 2008, Amsterdam, Netherlands. New York: ACM Press.

Hey, J., C. Newman, J. Sandhu, C. Daniels, J.-S. Hsu, and A.M. Agogino. 2007. Designing mobile digital library services for pre-engineering and technology literacy. International Journal of Engineering Education 23(3): 441-453, Special Issue on Mobile Technologies for Engineering Education.

Höllerer, T., and S. Feiner. 2004. Mobile augmented reality. In Telegeoinformatics: Location-Based Computing and Services (H. Karimi and A. Hammad, eds). London: Taylor & Francis Books.

Hoshi, Y. 2011. Towards the next generation of near-infrared spectroscopy. Philosophical Transactactions of the Royal Society A. Mathematical, Physical, and Engineering Sciences 369:4425-4439. Available at http://rsta.royalsocietypublishing.org/content/369/1955/4425.full.pdf.

Hull, K. 1990. Biological Rhythms and Shift Work. Military Applications of Circadian Rhythm Principles (PB91215905). Decision Science Consortium, Inc., Reston, Va. Available at http://www.ntis.gov/search/product.aspx?ABBR=PB91215905. Accessed September 19, 2012.

Huys, R., D. Braeken, and D. Prodanov. 2011. Bio-Hybrid Implant for Connecting a Neural Interface with a Host Nervous System. US Patent 2011/0257501 A1. Filed April 11.

Hynna, K.M., and K.A. Boahen. 2009. Nonlinear influence of T-channels in an in silico relay neuron. IEEE Transactions on Biomedical Engineering 56:1734.

Iancu, C., S. Hofmeyr, F. Blagojevic, and Y. Zheng. 2010. Oversubscription on multicore processors. 2010 IEEE International Symposium on Parallel & Distributed Processing (IPDPS).

IBM. 2012. From Big Bang to Big Data: ASTRON and IBM Collaborate to Explore Origins of the Universe. Press release. Available at http://www-03.ibm.com/press/us/en/pressrelease/37361.wss. Last Accessed on June 26, 2012.

Indiveri, G., B. Linares-Barranco, T.J. Hamilton, A. van Schaik, R. Etienne-Cummings, T. Delbruck, S.-C. Liu, P. Dudek, P. Häfliger, S. Renaud, J. Schemmel, G. Cauwenberghs, J. Arthur, K. Hynna, F. Folowosele, S. Saigh, T. Serrano-Gotarredona, J. Wijekoon, Y. Wang and K. Boahen. 2011. Neuromorphic silicon neuron circuits. Frontiers in Neuroscience 5(73):1-20.

Izydorczyk, J. 2010. Microprocessor scaling: What limits will hold? IEEE Computer 43(8):20-26.

James, F.O., C.D. Walker, and D.B. Boivin. 2004. Controlled exposure to light and darkness realigns the salivary cortisol rhythm in night shift workers. Chronobiology International 21(6):961-972.

Johns, M.W., A. Tucker, R. Chapman, K. Crowley, and N. Michael. 2007. Monitoring eye and eyelid movements by infrared reflectance oculography to measure drowsiness in drivers. Somnologie 11:234-242.

Khademhosseini, A., J.P. Vacanti, and R. Langer. 2009. Progress in tissue engineering. Scientific American 300(5):64-71.

King, A.C., G. Belenky, and H.P. Van Dongen. 2009. Performance impairment consequent to sleep loss: Determinants of resistance and susceptibility. Current Opinion in Pulmonary Medicine 15(6):559-564, doi:10.1097/MCP.0b013e3283319aad.

Kipke, D.R., J.C. Williams, J. Hetke, and P.C. Garell. 2011. Intracranial neural interface system. US Patent 7979105 B2. Filed June 12, 2009. Issued July 12, 2011.

Kirilina, E., A. Jelzow, A. Heine, M. Niessing, H. Wabnitz, R. Brühl, B. Ittermann, A.M. Jacobs, and I. Tachtsidis. 2012. The physiological origin of task-evoked systemic artifacts in functional near infrared spectroscopy. Neuroimage 61:70-81.

Koomey, J. 2007. Estimating Total Power Consumption by Servers in the U.S. and the World. Oakland, Calif.: Analytics Press. February 15.

Kurihara, K., and K. Tsukada. 2012. SpeechJammer: A System Utilizing Artificial Speech Disturbance with Delayed Auditory Feedback. CoRR. abs/1202.6106. Available at http://arxiv.org/abs/1202.6106. Accessed on June 29, 2012.

Lancet, 2009. Health effects of Ramadan. Lancet 374(9690):588, doi:10.1016/S0140-6736(09)61506-3.

Laundry, B., and R. Lees. 1991. Industrial accident experience of one company on 8- and 12-hour shift systems. Journal of Occupational Medicine: Official Publication of the Industrial Medical Association 33(8):903-906.

Lee, K., J. He, R. Clement, S. Massia, and B. Kim. 2004. Biocompatible benzocyclobutene (BCB)-based neural implants with micro-fluidic channel. Biosensors and Bioelectronics 20: 404-407.

Lerman, S.E., E. Eskin, D.J. Flower, E.C. George, B. Gerson, N. Hartenbaum, S.R. Hursh, and M. Moore-Ede. 2012. Fatigue risk management in the workplace. Journal of Occupational and Environmental Medicine 54(2):231-258.

Lieberman, H., and T. Selker. 2003. Agents for the user interface. In Handbook of Agent Technology. Cambridge, Mass.: MIT Press.

Lieberman, H. 1998. Integrating user interface agents with conventional applications. Pp. 39-46 in Proceedings of the Third International Conference on Intelligent User Interfaces (IUI '98). San Francisco, Calif. New York: ACM Press.

Lindeman, R.W., and N. Haruo. 2007. A classification scheme for multi-sensory augmented reality. Proceedings of the 2007 ACM Symposium on Virtual Reality Software and Technology, VRST '07, New York: ACM Press.

Linden, A., and J. Fenn. 2003. Understanding Gartner's Hype Cycles, Gartner Research R-20-1971. Available at http://www.ask-force.org/web/Discourse/Linden-HypeCycle-2003.pdf.

Liu, C.C., and M. Milrad. 2010. Guest editorial--One-to-one learning in the mobile and ubiquitous computing age. Educational Technology and Society 13(4):1-3.

Lo, C. 2012. Kinect evolved: Stroke recovery with Microsoft's motion sensor. 12 July. Available at http://www.hospitalmanagement.net/features/featurekinect-stroke-recovery-microsoft-motion-sensor/. Accessed September 19, 2012.

Mackay, W.E. 1998. Augmented reality: Linking real and virtual worlds: A new paradigm for interacting with computers. Proceedings of the Working Conference on Advanced Visual Interfaces, AVI '98. New York: ACM Press.

Maguire, L.P., T.M. McGinnity, B. Glackin, A. Ghani, A. Belatreche, and J. Harkin. 2007. Challenges for large-scale implementations of spiking neural networks on FPGAs. Neurocomputing 71:13.

Mankoff, J., D. Matthews, S.R. Fussell, and M. Johnson. 2007. Leveraging social networks to motivate individuals to reduce their ecological footprints. P. 87 in Proceedings of International Conference on System Sciences.

Manyika, James, Brad Brown, Jacques Bughin, Richard Dobbs, Charles Roxburgh, and Angela Hung Byers. 2011. Big Data: The Next Frontier for Innovation, Competition, and Productivity. McKinsey Global Institute. McKinsey & Company. May. Available at http://www.mckinsey.com/insights/mgi/research/technology_and_innovation/big_data_the_next_frontier_for_innovation.

Matsumoto, T., and S. Hashimoto. 2009. Pileus Internet umbrella: Tangible mobile interface of a lovely umbrella. Pp. 41-42 in Proceedings of the 3rd International Conference on Tangible and Embedded Interaction (TEI '09). ACM, New York, and Pileus, Tokyo.

Matthews, G., P.A. Desmond, and P.A. Hancock, eds. 2012. The Handbook of Operator Fatigue. Ashgate.

McGettrick, K., and M. O'Neill. 2006. Critical care nurses—Perceptions of 12-h shifts. Nursing in Critical Care 11(4):188-197.

Meenderinck, C., and B. Juurlink, 2009. (When) will CMPs hit the power wall? Euro-Par 2008 Workshops--Parallel Processing. Berlin: Springer-Verlag.

Milgram, P., and F. Kishino 1994. A taxonomy of mixed reality visual displays. IEICE Transactions on Information Systems E77-D(12):1321-1329.

Miller, J.C. 2010. Fatigue Effects and Countermeasures in 24/7 Security Operations. ASIS Foundation Research Council CRISP Report. Available from http://www.asisonline.org/foundation/CRISP_Fatigue Effects.pdf.

Miller, J.C. 2005. A Fatigue Check and for Mishap Investigations. Report to the USAF Research Lab. AFRL-HE-BR-TR-2005-0071. May.

Miller, G.A. 1956. The magical number seven, plus or minus two: Some limits on our capacity for processing information. Psychological Review 63:81.

Modha, D.S., and R. Singh. 2010. Network architecture of the long-distance pathways in the macaque brain. Proceedings of the National Academy of Sciences 107(30):13485.

Morgan, F., S. Cawley, B. McGinley, S. Pande, U. McDaid, B. Glackin, J. Maher, and J. Harkin. 2009. Exploring the evolution of NoC-based spiking neural networks on FPGAs. P. 300 in International Conference on Field Programmable Technology. Available at http://postgrad.ucc.ie/en/eedsp/Research/Papers/FMorganPapers/FMorganIEEE/F-MorganIEEE.pdf.

Morrison, A., A. Oulasvirta, P. Peltonen, S. Lemmela, G. Jacucci, G. Reitmayr, J. Näsänen, and A. Juustila. 2009. Like bees around the hive: A comparative study of a mobile augmented reality map. In Proceedings of CHI '09. New York: ACM Press.

National Academy of Sciences, National Academy of Engineering, and Institute of Medicine. 2007. Rising Above the Gathering Storm: Energizing and Employing America for a Brighter Economic Future. Washington, D.C.: The National Academies Press. Available at http://www.nap.edu/catalog.php?record_id=11463.

National Academy of Sciences, National Academy of Engineering, Institute of Medicine (NAS, NAE, IOM). 2010. Rising Above the Gathering Storm, Revisited: Rapidly Approaching Category 5. Washington, D.C.: The National Academies Press. Available at http://www.nap.edu/catalog.php?record_id=12999.

National Research Council (NRC). 1992. Time Horizons and Technology Investments. Washington, D.C.: National Academy Press.

National Research Council. 1997a. Tactical Displays for Soldiers: Human Factors Considerations. Washington, D.C.: National Academy Press.

National Research Council. 1997b. Flight to the Future: Human Factors in Air Traffic Control. Washington, D.C.: National Academy Press.

National Research Council. 2005. Interfaces for Ground and Air Military Robots: Workshop Summary. Tal Oron-Gilad, rapporteur. Washington, D.C.: The National Academies Press.

National Research Council. 2007. Human-Systems Integration in the System Development Process: A New Look. R.W. Pew and A.S. Mavor, eds. Washington, D.C.: The National Academies Press.

National Research Council. 2011. Health Care Comes Home: The Human Factors. Washington, D.C.: The National Academies Press.

Navarro, X., T.B. Krueger; N. Lago, S. Micera, T. Stieglitz, and P. Dario. 2005. A critical review of interfaces with the peripheral nervous system for the control of neuroprostheses and hybrid bionic systems. Journal of the Peripheral Nervous System 10(3):229-258, doi: 10.1111/j.1085-9489.2005.10303.x. September.

New, R. 2008. The Future of Magnetic Recording Technology. Available at http://asia.stanford.edu/events/spring08/slides402S/0410-Dasher.pdf.

Nickolls, J., and W.J. Dally. 2010. The GPU computing era. IEEE Micro 30:56. Available at http://sbel.wisc.edu/Courses/ME964/Literature/onGPUcomputingDally2010.pdf.

Norman, D.A. 1980. Twelve issues for cognitive science. Cognitive Science 4(1):1-32.

Norman, D.A. 1993. Things That Make the U.S. Smart. Cambridge, Mass.: Perseus Publishing.

Norman, D.A. 2011. Why Human Systems Integration Fails (and Why the University Is the Problem). Invited talk for the 30th anniversary of the Human-Systems Integration Board of the National Research Council, December 2, 2010, Washington, D.C. Available at http://www.jnd.org/dn.mss/why_human_systems_integration_fails_and_why_the_university_is_the_problem.html. Accessed June 29, 2012.

Normand, J.M., M. Servières, and G. Moreau. 2012. A new typology of augmented reality applications. In Proceedings of the 3rd Augmented Human International Conference (AH '12). New York, N.Y.: ACM Press.

Nuyujukian, P., J.M. Fan, V. Gilja, P.S. Kalanithi, C.A. Chestek, and K.V. Shenoy. 2011. Monkey models for brain-machine interfaces: The need for maintaining diversity. Proceedings of the 33rd Annual International Conference of the IEEE Engineering in Medicine and Biology Society, August 30-September 3, 2011, Boston, Mass.

Office of Technology Assessment, U.S. Congress. 1991. Biological Rhythms: Implications for the Worker. New Developments in Neuroscience (No. PB92117589). Washington, D.C.: U.S. Government Printing Office. Available at http://www.princeton.edu/~ota/ns20/alpha_f.html.

Olsson, T., E. Lagerstam, T. Kärkkäinen, and K. Väänänen-Vainio-Mattila. 2011. Expected user experience of mobile augmented reality services: A user study in the context of shopping centers. Journal of Personal and Ubiquitous Computing.

Olsson, J.A., and P. Häfliger. 2008. Mismatch reduction with relative reset in integrate-and-fire photo-pixel array. Pp. 277-280 in Proceedings of the Biomedical Circuits and Systems Conference. IEEE BioCAS Conference 2008, Baltimore, Md.

Park, D., T. Nam, and C. Shi. 2006. Designing an immersive tour experience system for cultural tour sites. Conference on Human Factors in Computing Systems (CHI 2006), Montreal, Canada.

Pasley, B.N., S.V. David, N. Mesgarani, A. Flinker, S.A. Shamma, N.E. Crone, R.T. Knight, and E.F. Chang. 2012. reconstructing speech from human auditory cortex. PLoS Biology 10(1):e1001251.

Paul, M.A., J.C. Miller, G. Gray, F. Buick, S. Blazeski, and J. Arendt. 2007. Circadian phase delay induced by phototherapeutic devices. Aviation, Space, and Environmental Medicine 78(7):645-652.

Paulos, E., M. Forth, S. Satchell, Y. Kim, P. Dourish, and J. Choi. 2008. Ubiquitous sustainability: Citizen science and activism. In Proceedings of Ubicomp '08 Workshops.

Pearson, M.J., A.G. Pipe, B. Mitchinson, K. Gurney, C. Melhuish, I. Gilhespy, and M. Nibouche. 2007. Implementing spiking neural networks for real-time signal-processing and control applications: A model-validated FPGA approach. IEEE Transactions on Neural Networks 18:1472.

Perez, C. 2002. Technological Revolutions and Financial Capital: The Dynamics of Bubbles and Golden Ages. Cheltenham, U.K.: Edward Elgar Publishing.

Pfeifer, R., J. Bongard, and S. Grand. 2007. How the Body Shapes the Way We Think: A New View of Intelligence. Cambridge, Mass.: MIT Press.

Piérard, C., M. Beaumont, M. Enslen, F. Chauffard, D.X. Tan, R.J. Reiter, A. Fontan, et al. 2001. Resynchronization of hormonal rhythms after an eastbound flight in humans: Effects of slow-release caffeine and melatonin. European Journal of Applied Physiology 85(1-2):144-150.

Raghu, S. 2010. Invention to Product: Processes and Time-Lines. Entrepreneurship for Physicists and Engineers.

Rahman, S.A., S. Marcu, C.M. Shapiro, T.J. Brown, and R.F. Casper. 2011. Spectral modulation attenuates molecular, endocrine, and neurobehavioral disruption induced by nocturnal light exposure. American Journal of Physiology-Endocrinology and Metabolism 300:E518-E527.

Rebsamen, B., C. Guan, H. Zhang, C. Wang, C. Teo, M.H. Ang, Jr., and E. Burdet. 2010. A brain controlled wheelchair to navigate in familiar environments. IEEE Transactions on Neural Systems and Rehabilitation Engineering 18(6):590-598.

Reeves, D.L., J. Bleiberg, T. Roebuck-Spencer, A.N. Cernich, K. Schwab, B. Ivins, A.M. Salazar, et al. 2006. Reference values for performance on the Automated Neuropsychological Assessment Metrics V3.0 in an active duty military sample. Military Medicine 171(10):982-994.

Reeves, D.L., K.P. Winter, J. Bleiberg, and R.L. Kane. 2007. ANAM® genogram: Historical perspectives, description, and current endeavors. Archives of Clinical Neuropsychology 22(Supplement 1, 0):15-37, doi:10.1016/j.acn.2006.10.013.

Richardson, A., C. Turnock, L. Harris, A. Finley, and S. Carson. 2007. A study examining the impact of 12-hour shifts on critical care staff. Journal of Nursing Management 15(8):838-846, doi:10.1111/j.1365-2934.2007.00767.x.

Rogers, E.M. 1962. Diffusion of Innovations. Glencoe, Ill.: Free Press.

Rogers, E.M. 1983. Diffusion of Innovations. New York: Free Press.

Rogers, Y., S. Price, G. Fitzpatrick, R. Fleck, E. Harris, H. Smith, C. Randell, H. Muller, C. O'Malley, D. Stanton, M. Thompson, and M. Weal. 2004. Ambient Wood: Designing new forms of digital augmentation for learning outdoors. Pp. 3-10 in Proceedings of Interaction Design and Children. New York: ACM Press.

Rolland, Y., F. Pillard, A. Klapouszczak, E. Reynish, D. Thomas, S. Andrieu, D. Rivière, and B. Vellas. 2007. Exercise program for nursing home residents with Alzheimer's disease: A 1-year randomized, controlled trial. First published online January 8, doi:10.1111/j.1532-5415.2007.01035.x.

Ros, E., E.M. Ortigosa, R. Agís, R. Carrillo, and M. Arnold. 2006. Real-time computing platform for spiking neurons (RTspike). IEEE Transactions on Neural Networks 17:1050.

Roschelle, J. 2003. Keynote paper: Unlocking the learning value of wireless mobile devices. Journal of Computer Assisted Learning 19(3):260-272.

Rothfarb, R.J. 2011. Science in the city AR: Using mobile augmented reality for science inquiry activities. ACM SIGGRAPH 2011 Posters (SIGGRAPH '11). New York: ACM Press.

Ruei-Zeng, L., and C. Hwan-You. 2008. Recent advances in three-dimensional multicellular spheroid culture for biomedical research. Biotechnology Journal 3(9-10):1285.

Rusu, M.I. 2007. New phase-change materials to achieve cognitive computer—Overview and future trends. International Conference on Transparent Optical Networks 4:287.

Ryokai, K., and A.M. Agogino. Off the paved paths: Exploring nature with a mobile augmented reality learning tool. Journal of Mobile HCI (IJMHCI). In press.

Sachlos, E., and D.T. Auguste. 2008. Embryoid body morphology influences diffusive transport of inductive biochemicals: A strategy for stem cell differentiation. Biomaterials 29:4471-4480.

Samaha, E., S. Lal, N. Samaha, and J. Wyndham. 2007. Psychological, lifestyle and coping contributors to chronic fatigue in shift-worker nurses. Journal of Advanced Nursing 59(3):221-232, doi:10.1111/j.1365-2648.2007.04338.x.

Schall, G., E. Mendez, E. Kruijff, E. Veas, S. Junghanns, B. Reitinger, and D. Schmalstieg. 2009. Handheld augmented reality for underground infrastructure visualization. Personal and Ubiquitous Computing 13(4):281-291.

Schemmel, J., J. Fieres, and K. Meier. 2008. Wafer-scale integration of analog neural networks. Pp. 431-438 in Proceedings of the IEEE International Joint Conference on Neural Networks, Hong Kong.

Schnell, T., J.E. Melzer, and S.J. Robbins. 2009. The cognitive pilot helmet: Enabling pilot-aware smart avionics. Proceedings of SPIE 7326:73260A-73260A-9, Special Issue Head- and Helmet-Mounted Displays XIV: Design and Applications.

Sefton-Green, J. 2003. Literature Review in Informal Learning with Technology Outside School. NESTA Futurelab, Bristol, U.K. Available at www.nestafuturelab.org/research/lit_reviews.htm.

Seo, J.-S., B. Brezzo, Y. Liu, B.D. Parker, S.K. Esser, R.K. Montoye, B. Rajendran, J.A. Tierno, L. Chang, D.S. Modha, and D.J. Friedman. 2011. A 45 nm CMOS neuromorphic chip with a scalable architecture for learning in networks of spiking neurons. Custom Integrated Circuits Conference.

Simon, H.A. 1971. Designing organizations for an information-rich world. Computers, Communication, and the Public Interest (M. Greenberger). Baltimore, Md.: Johns Hopkins Press.

Smith, L., S. Folkard, P. Tucker, and I. Macdonald. 1998. Work shift duration: A review comparing eight hour and 12 hour shift systems. Occupational and Environmental Medicine 55(4):217-229.

Soloway, E., W. Grant, R. Tinker, J. Roschelle, M. Mills, M. Resnick, R. Berg, and M. Eisenberg. 1999. Science in the palm of their hands. Communications of the ACM 42(8):21-26.

Son, I.-Y., and B. Yazici. 2005. Near infrared imaging and spectroscopy for brain activity monitoring. Pp. 341-372 in Advances in Sensing with Security Applications. NATO Security Through Sciences Series-A: Chemistry and Biology (J. Byrnes, ed.). Dordrecht, The Netherlands: Springer. Available at http://www.ecse.rpi.edu/~yazici/bio_book.pdf. Accessed August 2, 2012.

Thomson, J.A., J. Itskovitz-Eldor, S.S. Shapiro, M.A. Waknitz, J.J. Swiergiel, V.S. Marshall, et al. 1998. Embryonic stem cell lines derived from human blastocysts. Science 282:1145-1147.

Tucker, P., L. Smith, I. Macdonald, and S. Folkard. 1998. Shift length as a determinant of retrospective on-shift alertness. Scandinavian Journal of Work, Environment and Health 24(Supplement 3):49-54.

Upegui, A., C.A. Pena-Reyes, and E. Sanchez. 2005. An FPGA platform for on-line topology exploration of spiking neural networks. Microprocessors and Microsystems 29:211.

U.S. Code. 2008. Report to Congress on Server and Data Center Energy Efficiency. Public Law 109-431.

Veas, E.E., and E. Kruijff. 2010. Handheld devices for mobile augmented reality. In Proceedings of the 9th International Conference on Mobile and Ubiquitous Multimedia (MUM '10). Graz University of Technology, Austria. New York: ACM Press.

Vetter, R.J., R.H. Olsson III, J.F. Hetke, J.C. William, D. Pellinen, K.D. Wise, and D.R. Kipke. 2003. Silicon-substrate intracortical microelectrode arrays with integrated electronics for chronic cortical recording. Proceedings of the 25th Annual International Conference of the IEEE Engineering in Medicine and Biology Society, September 17-21 2003, Cancun, Mexico.

Wang, X.H., Y.N. Yan, Y.Q. Pan, Z. Xiong, H.X. Liu, B. Cheng, et al. 2006. Generation of three-dimensional hepatocyte/gelatin structures with rapid prototyping system. Tissue Engineering 12(1):83-90.

Welch, G., and G. Bishop. 1997. SCAAT: Incremental tracking with incomplete information. SIGGRAPH 97 Conference Proceedings. ACM SIGGRAPH, August 1997, Los Angeles, Calif.

West, S., M. Ahern, M. Byrnes, and L. Kwanten. 2007. New graduate nurses' adaptation to shift work: Can we help? Collegian (Royal College of Nursing, Australia) 14(1):23-30.

Whitaker Foundation. 2009. The Whitaker Foundation. Available at http://www.whitaker.org/home/the_whitaker_foundation. Accessed June 21, 2012.

White, S., and S. Feiner. 2010. Exploring interfaces to botanical species classification. Proceedings of the 28th International Conference on Human Factors in Computing Systems, April 10-15, 2010, Atlanta, Ga. New York: ACM Press.

Williamson, A.M., C.G.I. Gower, and B.C. Clarke. 1994. Changing the hours of shiftwork: A comparison of 8- and 12-hour shift rosters in a group of computer operators. Ergonomics 37(2):287-298.

Wolpaw, J., N. Birbaumer, D. McFarland, G. Pfurtscheller, and T. Vaughan. 2002. Brain-computer interfaces for communication and control. Clinical Neurophysiology 113:767-791.

Yu, T., and G. Cauwenberghs. 2010. Analog VLSI biophysical neurons and synapses with programmable membrane channel kinetics. IEEE Transactions on Biomedical Circuits and Systems 4:139.

Zhang, L., and T.J. Webster. 2009. Nanotechnology and nanomaterials: Promises for improved tissue regeneration. Nano Today 4(1):66-80, doi:10.1016/j.nantod.2008.10.014. February.

Zia, A., O. Erdogan, P.M. Belemijan, K. Jin-Woo, M. Chu, R.P. Kraft, J.F. McDonald, and K. Bernstein. 2009. Mitigating memory wall effects in high-clock-rate and multicore CMOS 3-D processor memory stacks. P. 108 in Proceedings of the IEEE 97.

Appendixes

Appendix A
Biographic Sketches of Committee Members

Hendrick W. Ruck (*Chair*) is CEO and president of the Human Performance Consulting Group, LLC (HPCG). Company accomplishments include advising the medical-network CEO on planning, visioning, and building patient-care innovation; enhancing applied research; growth in clinical trials; and initiation of translational research programs. Dr. Ruck served as associate director, special team, in the Office of Science and Technology Policy, where he led a White House team to bring education technology from academic and government laboratories to education and training settings in the United States. He served as director of Air Force Research Laboratory human effectiveness, where he led a 1,200-person research group in training methods and systems; system interface design technologies; physiologic, psychologic, and physical effects of extreme environments on individual and team performance; and personnel protection. Dr. Ruck received the Presidential Rank Award in 2007. He holds a PhD in applied (industrial/organizational) psychology, an MMS in management science, and a BS, all from the Stevens Institute of Technology.

Julie J.C.H. Ryan (*Vice Chair*) is associate professor and chair of engineering management and systems engineering at George Washington University. She holds a BS in humanities from the US Air Force Academy, an MLS in technology from Eastern Michigan University, and a DSc in engineering management from George Washington University. Dr. Ryan began her career as an intelligence officer in the US Air Force and the US Defense Intelligence Agency. After leaving government service, she continued to serve US national-security interests in positions in industry. Her interests are in information-security and information-warfare research. She was a member of the National Research Council Naval Studies Board from 1995 to 1998.

Alice M. Agogino (NAE) is the Roscoe and Elizabeth Hughes Professor of Mechanical Engineering and an affiliated faculty member of the University of California, Berkeley (UCB) Haas School of Business. She also directs the Berkeley Expert Systems Technology Laboratory and the Berkeley Instructional Technology Studio. She has served in a number of administrative positions at UCB, including associate dean of engineering and faculty assistant to the executive vice chancellor and provost in educational development and technology. She continues as principal investigator for the National Engineering Education Delivery System and the digital libraries of courseware in science, mathematics, engineering, and technology. She received a BS in mechanical engineering from the University of New Mexico (1975), an MS in mechanical engineering (1978) from UCB, and a PhD from the Department of Engineering-Economic Systems of Stanford University (1984). She is a member of the Association of Women in Science and received the National Science Foundation Director's Award for Distinguished Teaching Scholars in 2004. She served as member of the Committee on Women in Academic Science and

Engineering of the National Academies Committee on Science, Engineering, and Public Policy. She is a member of the National Academy of Engineering.

Debra Auguste is an assistant professor of biomedical engineering at the City College of New York. Previously she was an assistant professor of biomedical engineering in the School of Engineering and Applied Sciences of Harvard University and an assistant professor in the Department of Surgery of Harvard Medical School. Earlier, she was a postdoctoral associate at the Massachusetts Institute of Technology (MIT). Her interests include drug and gene delivery, targeted delivery, stimulus-sensitive materials, and scaffolds for tissue engineering. Dr. Auguste is the principal investigator on grants from the Office of Naval Research (ONR), the Defense Advanced Research Projects Agency (DARPA), the National Science Foundation (NSF), and the Juvenile Diabetes Research Foundation (JDRF). She is a recipient of various awards, including the NSF CAREER Award in 2011, the DARPA Young Faculty Award in 2009, the Percy Julien Award for Outstanding Scientist of the Year in 2008, the ONR Young Investigator Award in 2007, the JDRF Innovation Award in 2007, the 1930 Wallace Memorial Honorific Fellowship in 2003, and several fellowships. In addition, Dr. Auguste was named to the 50 Most Influential African Americans in Technology list in 2009. She received her SB in chemical engineering from MIT in 1999 and her PhD in chemical engineering from Princeton University in 2005.

Steven G. Boxer (NAS) is the Camille and Henry Dreyfus Professor of Chemistry at Stanford University. His research interests include model membranes, energy and electron transfer dynamics in photosynthetic reaction centers, electrostatics and dynamics in proteins, and excited-state dynamics in green fluorescent proteins. He is an elected fellow of the American Association for the Advancement of Science, the American Academy of Arts and Sciences, the Biophysical Society, and the Royal Society of Chemistry. In 2008, he was elected to the National Academy of Sciences. He won the Max Tishler Award for Tufts University in 2007 and the Earle K. Plyler Prize for Molecular Spectroscopy in 2008. Dr. Boxer holds a BS in chemistry from Tufts University and a PhD in physical and physical-organic chemistry from the University of Chicago.

Christopher C. Green is assistant dean for Asia Pacific of the Wayne State School of Medicine (SOM). He is also a clinical fellow and professor in neuroimaging and magnetic resonance imaging in the Department of Diagnostic Radiology and the Department of Psychiatry and Behavioral Neurosciences of SOM and the Detroit Medical Center (DMC). His medical specialties are brain imaging and forensic neurology, and his personal medical practice is in the differential diagnosis of neurodegenerative disease. He serves on many government advisory groups and private-sector corporate boards of directors. Immediately before his current position, he was executive director for emergent technology research for SOM and DMC. From 1985 through 2004, he was executive director for global technology policy and chief technology officer for General Motors Asia-Pacific Operations. His career at General Motors included positions as head of biomedical sciences research and executive director of the General Motors Research Laboratory for Materials and Environmental Sciences. His career with the Central Intelligence Agency extended from 1969 to 1985 as a senior division analyst and assistant national intelligence officer for science and technology. His PhD in neurophysiology is from the University of Colorado Medical School, and his MD is from the Autonomous City University in El Paso, Texas, and Monterey, Mexico, with honors. He also holds the National Intelligence Medal and is a fellow of the American Academy of Forensic Sciences.

Hendrik F. Hamann is currently a research manager for physical analytics in the Physical Sciences Department at the IBM T.J. Watson Research Center, Yorktown Heights, New York. In 1995 he joined JILA (Joint institute between the University of Colorado and NIST) as a research associate in Boulder, Colorado. During his tenure at JILA he developed novel near-field optical microscopes to study single molecules at high spatial resolution. Since 2001, he has led the Physical Analytics program in IBM Research, first as a research staff member and currently as a research manager. His current research interest includes nanoscale heat transfer and energy management of large-scale computing systems as well as novel applications of physical modeling to infrastructure. He has authored and co-authored more than 80 peer-reviewed scientific papers and holds over 55 patents and has over 35 pending patent applications. Dr. Hamann is an IBM master inventor and has served on governmental committees such as with the National Academy of Sciences and as an industrial advisor to universities. He is a member of the American Physical Society (APS), Optical Society of America (OSA), Institute of Electrical and Electronics Engineers (IEEE), and the New York Academy of Sciences. Dr. Hamann received a diploma in chemical physics (1992) and his PhD (1995) from the University of Göttingen, Germany.

James C. Miller is a human-factors consultant in San Antonio, Texas. He provides expertise to the Control Room Management Team of the Pipeline and Hazardous Materials Safety Administration of the U.S. Department of Transportation and supports applied psychophysiologic research in the U.S. Army Research Institute of Environmental Medicine. Dr. Miller was the founding director of the Human Environmental Research Center at the U.S. Air Force Academy (USAFA), Colorado Springs, Colorado. He also helped to design and then chaired the USAFA Institutional Review Board for the protection of human subjects in research from 1998 to 2000. In 2000, Dr. Miller helped to create the Air Force Research Laboratory's Warfighter Fatigue Countermeasures R&D Group at Brooks City-Base in San Antonio, Texas. Dr. Miller is a certificant of the Board of Certification in Professional Ergonomics and reviews applications for certification. He is the author of the book *Fatigue* in the *Controlling Pilot Error* series of McGraw-Hill (2001), a former founding associate editor of *Ergonomics in Design,* a former reviewer for *Aviation, Space, and Environmental Medicine,* and author of the report *Fatigue Effects and Countermeasures in 24/7 Security Operations* for the ASIS Foundation (2010). He is a former chair of the Department of Defense Human Factors Engineering Technical Advisory Group and an emeritus member of the Human Factors and Ergonomics Society and the Aerospace Medical Association. In 2007, he received the Henry L. Taylor Founder's Award for outstanding contributions in the field of aerospace human factors from the Aerospace Human Factors Association. Dr. Miller received his BA in analytic biology and his PhD in biology (environmental physiology) from the University of California, Santa Barbara.

Joanna Mirecki Millunchick is a professor of materials science and engineering and is affiliated with the Applied Physics Program and the Michigan Center for Theoretical Physics at the University of Michigan. Her general research interests involve manipulating matter on the nanoscale to enable the design of new electronic materials for optoelectronic and microelectronic applications. Her specific interests are in the materials and surface sciences of semiconductor thin-film nucleation and epitaxy, using a number of growth platforms, including molecular-beam epitaxy, chemical-vapor deposition, and ion-assisted deposition. A variety of characterization techniques are used to study structural properties (reflection high-energy electron diffraction, x-ray diffraction, transmission electron microscopy, and atomic-force microscopy), electronic properties (Hall and resistivity measurements), and optical properties (photoluminescence) of these films. Dr. Millunchick has received several awards, including the National Science Foundation CAREER Award, the Sloan Foundation Pre-Tenure Fellowship, and the John F. Ullrich Education Excellence Award from the University of Michigan. She received her BS in physics from DePaul University in Chicago in 1990 and her PhD in materials science and engineering from Northwestern University in Evanston in 1995.

Donald Norman (NAE) is a cofounder of the Nielsen Norman Group; a professor emeritus of the University of California, San Diego, where he served as chair of the Psychology Department and founder and chair of the Cognitive Science Department and Breed Professor of Design emeritus; and professor emeritus of electrical engineering and computer science of Northwestern University. He is a former vice president of Apple and a former executive of Hewlett Packard. Dr. Norman serves as an IDEO Fellow and is on company boards and advisory boards. He has been Distinguished Visiting Professor of Industrial Design at the Korea Advanced Institute of Science and Technology (KAIST). He has received honorary degrees from the University of Padua (Italy) and the Technical University of Delft (the Netherlands); the Lifetime Achievement Award from SIGCHI, the professional organization for computer–human interaction; and the Benjamin Franklin Medal in Computer and Cognitive Science from the Franklin Institute (Philadelphia). He is a member of the National Academy of Engineering and a fellow of the American Academy of Arts and Sciences, the Association for Computing Machinery, the American Psychological Association, the Association for Psychological Science, the Human Factors and Ergonomics Society, and the Design Research Society. He serves on the Board of Trustees of IIT's Institute of Design in Chicago. His books include numerous textbooks and monographs in psychology and cognitive science and, most recently, books on design: *The Design of Everyday Things, Things That Make Us Smart, Emotional Design,* and *Living with Complexity.*

Laurie Zoloth, a Charles Deering McCormick Professor of Teaching Excellence, is director of the Brady Program in Ethics and Civic Life at Weinberg College of Arts and Sciences at Northwestern University, and was the founding director of the Center for Bioethics, Science and Society at Northwestern University`s Feinberg School of Medicine. She teaches in the Medical Humanities and Bioethics Program, in the Jewish Studies program, and as a professor of religious studies. From 1995 to 2003, she was a founder and director of the Program in Jewish Studies of San Francisco State University. In 2011, she was elected vice president of the American Academy of Religion. In 2001, she was the president of the American Society for Bioethics and Humanities, she was a two-term member of its founding board, and she received its Distinguished Service Award in 2007. She was a founder and vice president of the Society for Jewish Ethics and is a current board member. She served two terms as a member of the National Aeronautics and Space Administration (NASA) National Advisory Council, the nation's highest civilian advisory board for NASA, for which she received the NASA National Public Service Award in 2005; the Executive Committee of the International Society for Stem Cell Research; and she was the founding chair of the Howard Hughes Medical Institute's Bioethics Advisory Board. She has also been on the founding national boards of the American Society for Bioethics and Humanities, the International Society for Stem Cell Research, the Society for Scriptural Reasoning, and NASA's International Planetary Protection Advisory Committee. In 2005, she was honored as the Graduate Theological Union's alumna of the year; and in 2009, she received Northwestern University`s most distinguished award for teaching. In 2011, she was named to the City of Evanston Environmental Board. Dr. Zoloth received her doctorate in social ethics from the Graduate Theological Union and an MA in Jewish Studies from Graduate Theological Union, The Center for Jewish Studies in May 1993; an MA in English from California State University (San Francisco State) in 1991; a BSN from the University of the State of New York in 1982; and a BA in women's studies from the University of California, Berkeley (Phi Beta Kappa and Cum Laude) in 1974.

Appendix B
Meetings and Speakers

MEETING 1
JANUARY 19-20, 2012
THE KECK CENTER OF THE NATIONAL ACADEMIES
WASHINGTON, D.C.

Committee Charge and Sponsor Expectations for Study
Greg Gordon, US Army

Biological Op Cycle Discussion
James Miller, Committee Member

Biomemetics Discussion
Hendrik Hamann, Committee Member

Embedded Computing Discussion
Julie Ryan, Vice Chair

Wearable Computing Discussion
Steven Boxer, Committee Member

MEETING 2
MARCH 8-9, 2012
THE KECK CENTER OF THE NATIONAL ACADEMIES
WASHINGTON, D.C.

Out-of-the-Box Science for Human Performance Modification
Dylan Schmorrow, Deputy Director, Human Performance, Training and BioSystems Research Directorate
Office of the Assistant Secretary of Defense (OSD)

Sponsor Discussion
Greg Gordon
U.S. Army

Operator State Characterization Using Neurophysiological Measures
Thomas Schnell, Associate Professor
University of Iowa

Brain Computer Interface – Current Status, Future Prospects
Jonathon Wolpaw, Chief, Laboratory of Nervous Systems Disorders
Wadsworth Center, New York

Advanced Neurotechnologies for Science & Healthcare
Daryl Kipke, Professor, Department of Biomedical Engineering
University of Michigan

Technologies for Fatigue Detection and Management
Adam Fletcher, Executive Director
Integrated Safety Support, Australia

Fatigue, Jetlag and Shiftlag in RCAF Operations
Michel Paul, Defence Scientist
Defence Research and Development, Canada

Emergent Technosciences and Human Augmentation
Ana Viseu, Assistant Professor
York University, Canada
Universidade de Coimbra, Portugal

Reshaping the Human Condition – Exploring Human Enhancement
Jan Staman, Director
Ira van Keulen, Senior researcher Technology Assessment
Rathenau Institute, The Netherlands

MEETING 3
MARCH 29-30, 2012
THE BECKMAN CENTER OF THE NATIONAL ACADEMIES
IRVINE, CA

Biological Approaches to Improve Musculoskeletal Tissue Healing after Disease, Injury & Aging
Johnny Huard, Director
Stem Cell Research Center, University of Pittsburgh

Bioethics Discussion
Hank Greely, Deane F. and Kate Edelman Johnson, Professors of Law
Stanford University

Human Genetic Modification – Therapy and Enhancement
Theodore Friedmann, Chair, Gene Doping Expert Group
World Anti-Doping Agency
University of California at San Diego

Sponsor Perspectives
Greg Gordon, US Army
Mark Sulcoski, US Army

Expertise, Skill Learning and Human Development Across Domains
A. Mark Williams, Professor
Liverpool John Moores University
Research Institute for Sport and Exercise Sciences, UK

Tissue Engineering and Regenerative Medicine
Rui Luis Reis, Director
3B's Research Group, Biomaterials, Biodegradables and Biomimetics
University of Minho, Portugal

Introduction to Nanotechnology & Nanomedicines
Theresa Allen, Professor of Pharmacology
University of Alberta, Canada

Augmented Cognition and Wearable Computing
Thad Starner, Contextual Computing Group
Georgia Tech

Appendix C
Acronyms and Abbreviations

AAAS	American Association for the Advancement of Science
AR	augmented reality
ASIC(s)	application-specific integrated circuit
BCI	brain–computer interface
CPU	central processing unit
EEG	electroencephalography
FPGA	field-programmable gate arrays
GPU	general-purpose processors
HPM	human performance modification
IT	information technology
MAR	mobile augmented reality
NN	neural network
SNN	spiking neural network

Appendix D
Contextual Issues

THE TECHNOLOGY ECOSYSTEM

Technology does not exist in a vacuum. For advances to occur, there must be an ecosystem of supporting elements, including basic science, engineering know-how, materials, energy, and imagination.

The concept of a technology ecosystem is portrayed in Figure D-1. The interaction of all the portrayed elements is important for the development of technological innovations or advances in existing applications. This concept is important because each element can influence the success or failure of a technological advance. Thus, considering the future of a technology or a class of capabilities must take all the elements into account.

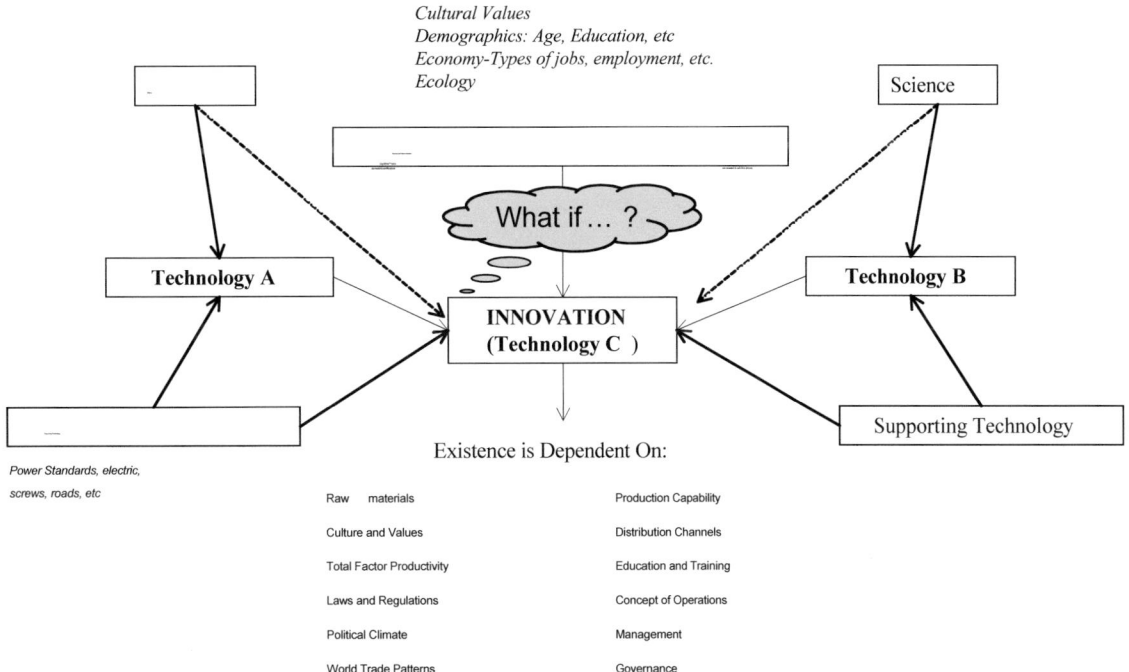

FIGURE D-1 The technology ecosystem.

Time is an intriguing and difficult element to consider in the context of a technology ecosystem. Time-related issues include time in existence, time to create, and time to innovate. Those all affect the richness and turmoil of an ecosystem.

- *Time in existence.* How long have the basic technological components been in existence? Technological components that have been in existence for a long time have the benefit of an existing support ecosystem: people who understand the technology and the science, existing applications, existence of manufacturers and support services, and other systemic elements. Newer technologies suffer in that fewer people understand the technology or the science and there are few manufacturers and support services.
- *Time to create.* How long does it take to make one instantiation of a new technology? In the case of complex systems that require the integration of many physical parts, such as a B-2 bomber, manufacture takes a long time. In the case of complex systems that require the integration of many logical parts, such as software, but not many physical parts, the finished product can go out on the market more quickly. The time it takes to make one of something affects an observer's opportunity to observe: faster products are harder to observe in production but easier to observe in distribution. The observation opportunities and speed of creation may influence imagining of moving technologies toward new uses.
- *Time to innovate.* The speed of innovation in the technology ecosystem may be tightly coupled to the nature of the particular technology. If the speed is fast, predictions of innovation can be easier than if it is slow. For example, many people are reasonably familiar with Moore's law, which makes it fairly easy to predict cycle times in computer systems. Predicting a cycle time for innovation in other industries is a little more difficult.

TECHNOLOGY FORECASTING

The committee describes here some aspects of technology forecasting that were applied for this report. The definition of a "successful" technology is important. Many technologies are being discovered and developed every day, but "useful" or "successful" technologies solve important and relevant problems in an economically viable way (whether for a commercial or a defense application). Given that definition and as depicted in Figure D-2, the challenge for technology forecasting comes from the fact that whether a technology is useful or not can change drastically while it is being developed. Consequently, technology forecasting is not just a matter of "labeling" and assessing maturity. It is a difficult and iterative task in which the environment constantly changes. The situation is like that of a moving target: a technology has to be constantly reassessed to permit understanding of whether it can provide a useful function at a future intersection point.

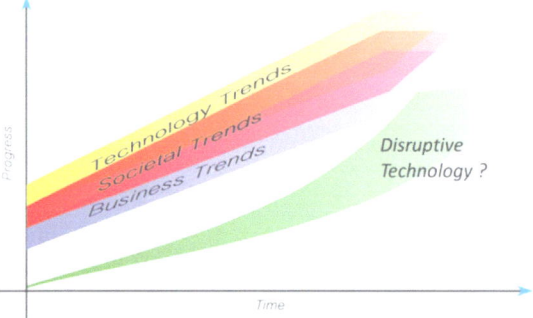

FIGURE D-2 Technology forecasting.

Generally, the usefulness of a technology will depend on the overall technology environment or ecosystem, but societal and business trends are also important. It is not uncommon for an application of a technology to change as it is being developed. For example, although energy-efficient light bulbs were developed to reduce energy consumption, they were first used in places where the high cost of changing a light bulb would provide enough incentive to use the more durable energy-efficient light bulbs. The general technology environment is important because relevant applications require integration of several technologies into a system. The availability of the other (enabling) technologies changes over time as well. Often, new and initially superior technologies will be outpaced by continued progress of existing ones. Other technologies can emerge, often for other markets, and make an existing technology suddenly obsolete or nonviable. Societal trends and the political environment are important, especially for human performance modification (HPM) technologies. The effect of the political environment on the development of controversial fields such as stem-cell research or nuclear energy technologies can be drastic and should not be underestimated.

Clearly, the longer it takes to develop a new technology, the less certain the likelihood of success is. One way to assess the time horizon and the technology potential is to look at the "product" lifetime and effect once the technology has been developed (NRC, 1992). Evidently, the time horizon for technology development depends on the product lifetime: a product with a longer lifetime can afford a longer time for development.

Generally, it can be useful to distinguish between two development approaches, and this can help in understanding both the potential and the required development time of a particular technology. As depicted in Figure D-3, one might want to distinguish between a "forward-based" and a "reverse-based" approach. A forward-based approach is typically based on a core technology or research and is exploratory. Basic research has to be carried out to investigate fundamentals of the science that underlies a technology before it can be developed and brought to market. In this scenario, market and products are often being developed after the core technology has been proved and is well under way to being developed. In contrast, a reverse approach is more opportunistic: one looks first at the application and the market opportunity and then finds often-existing technologies, which might need only to be assembled or integrated into a working system.

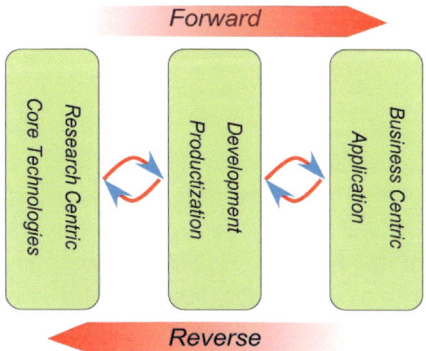

FIGURE D-3 Technology development approaches.

The relevance of that rather simplistic categorization is that the time horizon for forward-dominated approaches can be different from that for reverse-dominated approaches. Although most technology development is a combination of both approaches and changes over time, particularly as the technology matures, the time horizon in a forward-dominated approach can easily exceed 20 years. Such cases often involve high-risk projects that have unpredictable but potentially game-changing outcomes.

An example of a more forward-dominated approach is the development of near-field technologies for thermally assisted recording in magnetic hard disk drives. This technology allows boosting storage capacity by locally heating the magnetic media and thereby easing the recording process. The technology has been under development for more than 15 years and is projected to be complete in 2014-2015 (NRC, 1992). Near-field physics and engineering were pioneered in the 1970s and 1980s. Initial laboratory experiments demonstrated the viability of the technology for thermally assisted magnetic recording in 1995 and 2005 (New, 2008; Betzig et al., 1992), but the technology required much additional basic research and development to gain understanding of the underlying physics of the recording processing and the manufacturing process. In addition, throughout the development process, alternative technologies had emerged, such as perpendicular recording and improved magnetoresistive sensors. The alternatives could increase the storage density by different means, and this constantly changed the performance target for thermally assisted recording. Another example of forward-based approaches is the development of high-dielectric-constant materials to reduce gate leakage of a transistor, which took much more than 15 years.

In a reverse-dominated approach, the time horizon is much shorter—about 2-10 years—and the outcome is more predictable. This approach is "system-centric" with an eye toward a specific application. Most development and research work in industry is in this category. An example of a classical reverse approach is an improved windshield-washer nozzle that exploits hydrodynamic instabilities to distribute cleaning fluid on a windshield more evenly (Raghu, 2010). The full development cycle of the technology took less than 3 years and included a clever design of a bistable twin jet nozzle that could be adapted to a standard windshield fluid distribution system.

These examples are meant to provide support for the following notions:

- Forward-based approaches are less likely to be successful within the period that this report concerns, 15 years.
- It seems to be more likely that future HPM applications will be realized with a reverse-dominated approach that uses technologies that are off-the-shelf or in the late stages of development.
- Although forward-based approaches can result in the biggest "surprise", the vast variety of possible HPM applications coming from reverse-based, short-term development approaches could be as much a source of surprises as groundbreaking discoveries in a specific field.

There is an additional reason to pay careful attention to reverse-dominated approaches, based on common technology development models (Raghu, 2010; Perez, 2002). These models show that a typical technology cycle is triggered in a first phase by an initial discovery, followed by frenzy or hype, which results in a crash (Linden, 2003). The time between the discovery and the crash is around 30–50 years; this has been repeatedly observed in the history of technology. The crash is followed by a longer second phase, which is characterized by a slower but systematic adaptation of the technology, in which reverse-dominated technology-development approaches are favored. Although HPM involves a variety of technologies, the models suggest that the current HPM research environment resembles the second phase.

CULTURAL ISSUES

Cultural issues can be problematic with respect to both the understanding and the use of technologies. One issue is the approach to the development of technology. Another is the normalization of the use of technology. And a third is the interface between cultural norms and human performance. Layered on those issues is the cultural acceptability of copying innovation—what some might call theft of intellectual property.

The cultural values of a group can affect how technology is developed. Important cultural elements include respect for elders, the question of individuality versus community, and the cultural acceptance of failure. Cultures that place great value on seniority and deference to age tend to develop technologies more linearly and incrementally and in accordance with accepted practices. Innovation is difficult in such cultures. Conversely, cultures that accept and celebrate individuality tend to generate radical innovations that depart, sometimes dramatically, from accepted approaches and development structures. Cultures that view failure without shame as a natural potential result of risk-taking also tend to spawn more radical innovations; cultures that value team identities and view failure as a shameful state tend not to spawn radical innovations.

The normalization of the use of technology can affect the development of technologies. Some cultures, such as the Amish, specifically exclude some technologies from their lifestyle (Amish Heartland, 2012). Others adapt technologies in ways that the technology developers never envisioned. One can visualize this as a continuum of technology adoption and adaptation, and it has been the subject of much study, most notably by Rogers, who developed the concept of innovation diffusion (Rogers, 1962; Rogers, 1983). A study of Internet-adoption attitudes by female academic faculty in Saudi Arabian colleges illustrated the cultural barriers that can influence the adoption and development of technologies (Al-Kahtani et al., 2005-2006):

> There are sharp differences in the perceptions of elements of Saudi society . . . as to the potential use of the Internet. The more conservative elements of the society see more danger and shortcomings in Internet access than benefit. The members who are focused on new knowledge, such as the science faculty, are less likely to see the Internet as a danger and more likely to see it as a powerful tool for work enhancement.

The interface between cultural norms and human performance can present both challenges and opportunities. For example, the month-long fast of Ramadan in Islam has been shown to affect the biological health of participants (Lancet, 2009). The requirement for periodic religious practices during normal daily activities may affect human performance adversely. For example, depending on the geographic latitude and the season, it is possible for the first morning prayer in Islam to start as early as about 3 a.m. and the evening prayer as late as about 9 p.m. around the summer solstice. Daily participation in both prayers may lead to cumulative fatigue (Al-Kahtani et al., 2005-2006).

Finally, different cultures have different tolerances for or levels of acceptance of copying other people's work. In some cultures, copying innovations and technologies is not only accepted but rewarded. In other cultures, it is illegal. Interactions between those cultures can provide both the opportunity for tense geopolitical relationships and an environment for the development of advanced technologies that discourage copying.

MYTH-BUSTING

Predicting the future has never been easy, but there are many examples of the realization of science fiction, perhaps because it is not far from existing technology. Humans have always wanted to be better, smarter, and faster and to live longer—HPM is not new. Furthermore, multiple studies, not unlike the current one, have attempted to predict the future of HPM, so the obvious question is, how well did they do?[1]

In 2006, the American Association for the Advancement of Science (AAAS) published *Human Enhancement and the Means of Achieving It* (AAAS, 2006). Although that was only 6 years ago, it is instructive to look at some of the technologies highlighted in that study and where they are today. In the field of "artificial organs/implants", Bion devices, which electrically stimulate muscles, are highlighted. They are being used to treat arthritis but have the potential for

---

[1] The 1988 National Research Council report on human performance enhancement that discussed Department of Defense work on extrasensory perception, neurolinguistic programming, time travel, and "warrior monks" indicates how quickly plausible HPM "technologies" change. See NRC, 1988. *Enhancing Human Performance: Issues, Theories, and Techniques*, National Academy Press, Washington, D.C.. Available at http://www.nap.edu/openbook.php?isbn=0309037921.

performance enhancement. They appear to be in continuing studies, but not commercial products, although they were described in considerable detail 10 years ago. In the field of "interfacing with computers and technology", the report highlights brain implants at Brown University that are being developed by Cyberkinetics, now a part of BrainGate. The work was greeted with enormous interest and press attention; although it is fascinating and is still receiving press attention (for example, a recent dramatic movie showed a stroke victim moving an artificial arm and getting a drink), it remains largely a subject of research, not something that will affect the market (in this case, for rehabilitation) soon. In the field of nanotechnology, the report describes respirocytes, reputed to be able to "deliver 236 times more oxygen per unit volume than natural blood cells," in principle a tool for enhancing performance under extreme conditions (Freitas, 1996). The "device" was and still is hypothetical—something envisioned and not real. The 236-times enhancement of oxygen capacity is based on a calculation of something that does not exist.

These examples, a substantial fraction of the predictions of what would enhance human performance in a 2006 analysis, provide a cautionary note (AAAS, 2006). The remarkable pictures of a woman who has suffered a severe stroke and is using a brain implant to lift a water bottle and take a sip are dramatic evidence of progress, but practical technology, applicable to the battlefield, appears very unlikely. Any invasive device or chemical or biologic intervention that uses the tools of nanotechnology requires many years of development and testing, and genuinely disruptive technologies are, by their nature, unpredictable.

Perhaps the largest change is the emergence of bioengineering as a high-profile discipline that marries many fields of basic science, medicine, and engineering. The seeds planted by the Whitaker Foundation in the early 1980s have blossomed in many new university departments throughout the United States, and similar entities have rapidly emerged all over the world (Whitaker Foundation, 2009). This way of thinking about biological systems and ultimately humans is different from traditional biology or medicinal chemistry or from more traditional engineering fields, such as biomechanics. Large international consortia are focusing on building interfaces between tissues and devices, often computers. New treatments will emerge from the efforts, but probably not suddenly, and some of the results will be used to enhance human performance. The examples noted here suggest that it is easy to be seduced by dramatic visuals, and it is unlikely that one will be blind-sided by entirely new approaches.

CONCLUDING THOUGHTS

Technology development and adoption are messy, human processes that are resistant to clean predictability. There are methods for peering into the uncertain future to glimpse the potential, but the reality of human social existence affects the eventual actuality. Any effort to predict technologies must take into account not just the state of the science but also the state of humanity.